A History of United States Naval Aviation Medical Research During World War II

A HISTORY OF UNITED STATES NAVAL AVIATION MEDICAL RESEARCH DURING WORLD WAR II

Compiled by
Aviation Branch, Research Division
Bureau of Medicine and Surgery
Navy Department

1 June 1946

Reprinted by
Biological Sciences Division
Office of Naval Research

1 December 1975

TABLE OF CONTENTS

TABLE OF CONTENTS -

TABLE OF CONTENTS -

TABLE OF CONTENTS -

A

HISTORY OF UNITED STATES NAVAL AVIATION MEDICAL RESEARCH DURING WORLD WAR II

Compiled by

Aviation Branch, Research Division
Bureau of Medicine and Surgery
Navy Department

1 JUNE 1946

I. General Information

Aviation medical research began as a separate entity in the Navy in November, 1939, when Commander John R. Poppen, (MC), USN, reported to Chief, Bureau of Aeronautics to establish a Medical Research Section. Shortly thereafter, Commander Eric Liljencrantz, MC-V(S), USNR, was assigned to this section. The earliest work was concerned with problems of personnel selection and training, with visual problems and with the general hygiene and physiological problems of flying.

In March, 1941, Lieutenant Commander Leon D. Carson, (MC), USN, reported to this section and was assigned to the study of physiological requirements at higher altitudes, oxygen equipment, special visual problems of flying, accelerative stresses, and protection of flying personnel against cold and other hazards and stresses of flying.

By December, 1941, excellent liaison had been established with the Army Air Forces' research activities and with such civilian organizations as the National Research Council and the National Defense Research Committee. A subsection of psychologists and statisticians under the direction of Lieutenant Commander John G. Jenkins, H-V(S), USNR, had been set up to formulate and administer the selection and training program for aviation personnel. Major attention was being directed toward development of the Altitude Training Program at principal Air Training Centers and toward specifications for Altitude Chambers for research and indoctrination. Visual problems were being studied by Lieutenant Commander Carson who was also developing a new type of flying goggle.

Work continued under the jurisdiction of the Bureau of Aeronautics until October, 1942, when the research group of psychologists was transferred to the Division of Aviation Medicine of the Bureau of Medicine and Surgery; in September, 1943, the remaining activities and personnel of the section were transferred to the Research Division of the Bureau of Medicine and Surgery, with liaison officers assigned from the Bureau of Medicine and Surgery to the Flight Division under the Deputy Chief of Naval Operations, and to the Military Requirements Division under Chief, Bureau of Aeronautics. Captain Poppen and Lieutenant Commander Carson were the heads of this Section while it was under the Bureau of Aeronautics.

In 1942, Commander Liljencrantz became the first head of the Aviation Branch, Research Division, Bureau of Medicine and Surgery. After his death in November, 1942, this position was held by Lieutenant Commander Alfred Eyer, (MC), USN, until July, 1943. Subsequent heads of this Branch were Commander Wilbur Kellum, (MC), USN, from July to September, 1943, and Commander Carson from September, 1943, to April, 1944.

In April, 1944, Captain John H. Korb, (MC), USN, became head of the Aviation Branch, Research Division, Bureau of Medicine and Surgery and has continued in that capacity to the present time.

The objectives of Aviation Medical Research continue now as originally stated in September, 1943: "To apply results of Aviation Medical Research to problems of flying to (a) increase safety of flying, (b) to increase flying efficiency, and (c) to select and train personnel physically and psychologically qualified to fly. The Aviation Medical Research Section does not engage in actual research; it initiates and directs research effort toward the solution of problems of personnel engaged in military flying. These problems are, essentially, those of adaptation of man to the conditions and the environment of flight and are imposed by the environment itself and by the airplane."

II. Activities Engaged in Aviation Medical Research

The following activities have been active in conducting aviation medical research in the Navy:

1. School of Aviation Medicine, NAS, Pensacola, Florida

2. Naval Medical Research Institute, National Naval Medical Center, Bethesda, Maryland

3. Aero Medical Department, Naval Air Experimental Station, Naval Air Material Center, Philadelphia, Pennsylvania

4. Medical Field Research Laboratory, Camp Lejeune, North Carolina

5. Medical Research Department, U. S. Submarine Base, New London, Connecticut

6. Naval Air Training Bases, Corpus Christi, Texas

7. U. S. Naval Air Stations at San Diego, California; Alameda, California; Seattle, Washington; Norfolk, Virginia; Quonset Point, Rhode Island; Miami, Florida; Vero Beach, Florida; Jacksonville, Florida; and Anacostia, D. C.

8. U. S. Marine Corps Air Station, Cherry Point, North Carolina

In addition to the above, informal research was conducted at other naval activities and research of interest to the Navy was conducted at Army and civilian laboratories in the United States and in the allied countries.

III. Research Accomplishments in Specific Fields

In the discussion of specific research which follows, no attempt has been made to be all-inclusive in the matters of projects completed, personnel involved, etc. Rather, attempt has been made to make a general over-all summary of the accomplishments of Naval Aviation Medical Research during the war years, referring especially to the research projects conducted under Branch I, Research Division, Bureau of Medicine and Surgery, with supplementary reference to projects conducted under other Branches of the Research Division, to TED projects of the Bureau of Aeronautics, and to projects initiated and conducted by local activities.

A Bibliography of the research projects cited is appended to this history. There specific titles, dates and authors of reports may be found.

A. ACCELERATION

G-Suits

As early as 1932, Poppen conducted studies on the effects of acceleration and on protective measures against these effects. Such studies were first carried on in collaboration with the Fatigue Laboratory at Harvard. Subsequently, investigations were conducted at the Naval Aircraft Factory in Philadelphia. Through experiments using dogs, a compression belt was developed to provide support to the abdominal area as a means of preventing blood pooling in the splanchnic vessels. In 1939, a complete air suit with provisions for compression of the splanchnic area and lower extremities was developed and flight tested but was not considered successful enough for adoption. In 1940, a Toronto group developed a water pressure suit which was considered to be impractical for service use chiefly because of its bulk. In 1941, Ferwerda, in collaboration with the Berger Brothers Company, made a pulsatile-pressure suit. About the same time, the Moeller-Carson Gradient Pressure suit was developed. Both of the last mentioned two suits were flight-tested at Anacostia and Cecil Field, Florida in 1942. These proved to be effective in preventing blackout and grayout in maneuvers but definitely required further improvements. Because of difficulties encountered in producing adequate air-pumping devices, the pulsatile-pressure suit was rejected and the gradient pressure suit was made the object of further investigation.

In 1943, gradient pressure suits were delivered to combat squadrons for operational testing. Although pilots at first were enthusiastic about these suits, it was later found that they were still too cumbersome and impractical for universal service. However, a few of the suits were retained by the Navy and they were fairly widely used by the Army Air Forces.

In 1943, Clark and Wood at the Mayo Foundation developed an arterial occlusion suit which was tested and subsequently rejected.

In 1944, Schroeder conducted extensive tests in the Pacific on the gradient pressure suits. As a result of formulating the necessary requirements to make such equipment practical and acceptable, a single pressure suit was evolved from a modification of the old three-way gradient pressure suit. This suit was again modified by Moeller and Carson, was flight-tested at Eglin Field and was adopted by the Army Air Forces, although the Navy still considered it too bulky for universal use.

During the years 1941 to 1944, Clark and Berger worked on various models of suits. One model was intended to be a coverall type designed to enclose the necessary compression bladders while another model was to be a cut-out skeleton type comprised of isolated cuffs. The skeleton suit was endorsed by the Army Air Forces while the coverall suit, with modifications, was adopted by the Naval Air organization.

To quote from Commodore Adams' report on this development: "From the foregoing it is apparent that many individuals and organizations have participated in studies and tests relating to the development of the anti-G suit equipment. The Navy has been a pioneer and has assumed an active leadership in these studies. It has cooperated with the Army and other interested workers, in connection with these accomplishments. It is interesting to observe the difficulties that must be overcome in finally arriving at a practical and acceptable product of this kind, even though the scientific principles involved are entirely understood. It further demonstrates the importance of coordinating actual field studies (flight-testing) under operating conditions, with laboratory studies and commercial development. Early in the course of these studies a plan for circumventing blood pooling in splanchnic areas and lower extremities was recognized as the most direct approach in overcoming blackout and grayout from gravity stress. To convert this knowledge into an acceptable garment, and to develop reliable valve mechanisms of an automatic type for use with the appliance has taken a period of years. In view of the Navy's position with regard to these developments, the final accomplishment is one which may well be viewed with pride."

Other Studies

In September, 1945, Burt at Pensacola under Project X610 prepared an Annotated Bibliography on the Physiological Effects of Acceleration in Aircraft, comprising a listing of classified reports not otherwise available.

Research on acceleration is continuing at various service and civilian activities. Human centrifuge units will be in operation at Pensacola and Philadelphia for further investigation of the problem. Suggestions have been made for constructing monorail devices for more closely approximating conditions which will obtain in the extremely high speed aircraft envisioned for the future.

B. CLOTHING

General Survey

During the war, it became necessary to develop a great number of items of clothing for the protection of naval aviators against cold. The Navy expended considerable effort in the development of electrically-heated clothing. Most of the early work on this subject was carried out at the Industrial Hygiene Research Laboratory, National Institute of Health, under contract to the Bureau of Aeronautics. This work consisted primarily of an evaluation of the limitations of electrically-heated suits developed by several manufacturers; Colvinex, General Electric, Wolardarski, Thermo-equipment, and others. It was found that the standard Colvinex suit is adequate for long exposures at temperatures down to 0°F., while the standard Navy Shearling with unheated gloves and boots is adequate for exposure down to 20°F. For use at lower temperatures, electrically-heated gloves and boots are required. The Colvinex and Shearling remain the Standard Navy gear for cold weather although newer types of electrically-heated suits, alpaca-lined unheated suits, etc., have been used to some extent since 1945. In the latter part of the war, most of the test work for winter flight gear was carried out at the Naval Medical Research Institute and Naval Air Experimental Station, Philadelphia. (Projects X639 and X711).

The development of clothing for use in tropical climates was not particularly emphasized by Naval Aviation Medical Activities. A very satisfactory summer flying suit, made of nylon, was developed, but the extensive test program associated with the heavy winter gear was not required. One feature of the nylon suit which required considerable investigation, (conducted especially at the Naval Medical Research Institute), was the "inflammability" of nylon fabric and its flash-burn protection. It was determined that nylon may be considered a "non-inflammable" material in that it does not support combustion but reacts to heat only by melting. If weight, weave, and other factors are identical, cotton, silk, linen, and nylon appear to offer approximately equal protection against flash-burns.

Fundamental work on cooling the body during exposure to water of various temperatures was carried on at the Naval Medical Research Institute in Project X189. These studies added impetus to the development of a quick-donning anti-exposure suit for use by airmen in the event that ditching at sea became necessary. This suit was developed jointly by representatives of the Naval Medical Research Institute; Research Division, Bureau of Medicine and Surgery; Equipment and Materials Branch, Bureau of Aeronautics; and Military Requirements Division, Bureau of Aeronautics. In 1945, all planes flying over water that was expected to be below a certain critical temperature (70°F.) were equipped with suits of this type.

The disadvantages of attempting to don an exposure suit in the critical moments of ditching led to attempts to develop a suit appropriate for continuous wear, i.e., one permeable to water vapor and imperable to liquid water. Such a suit was designed at the Naval Medical Research Institute but was not issued to the service in any great quantity.

Among other items of special protective clothing, body armor devised for protection against anti-aircraft fragments was outstanding. The Research Division, Bureau of Medicine and Surgery, was responsible for the design and development of the aviator's nylon "flak suit", the "Doron" armored life jacket, and others, and successfully carried out the necessary administrative work to adoption by the naval service.

Other items of research pertaining to clothing which might be mentioned are the determination of the protection against ultra-violet light afforded by various fabrics, the determination of skin sensitivity to various fabrics, etc. In these categories, developments applied to the service at large rather than to aviation exclusively.

Specific Projects

Under Project X189, personnel at the Naval Medical Research Institute worked on the development of protective clothing for subjects immersed in cold water. Various trial models of immersion suits were made and sent to the Fleet for testing and evaluation. In addition, experiments were conducted on the reactions of human subjects to cooling and on the physiological effects of immersion. Work on this project is still continuing.

At the Naval Medical Research Institute under Project X227, Margolis and Shelesnyak developed a nylon "flak suit" for use by aviation personnel. This suit weighs approximately 19 pounds and consists of three units, (front, back, and apron), which may be worn as a complete unit or in various combinations of the individual parts. Unbonded nylon is used for penetration resistance, affording an area of protection of about seven square feet. This jacket, which integrates well with the pilot's flight gear and restraining harness can be instantly jettisoned with a single release strap.

Webster and Corey, Biodynamics Branch, Research Division, Bureau of Medicine and Surgery, under Project X640, designed an armored Navy summer flying jacket, weighing four pounds and utilizing a glass-fabric-plastic laminate, commonly called "Doron", which is inserted as plates in pockets of the jacket to afford maximum protection to the vital organs of the wearers. This jacket was found to resist the impact of .38 and .45 caliber revolver bullets, and the Thompson and Reising submachine guns, all fired from a distance of 15 feet; and to be effective against 20 mm. bursts, similar fragments, and against bayonets. This jacket is extremely light and comfortable and affords great ease of movement. This jacket was not formally adopted by the Bureau of Aeronautics before the end of the war, but was officially adopted by the Bureau of Ships for the Submarine Service.

C. DENTISTRY

Specific Projects

In May 1943, Restarski and Gersh at the Naval Medical Research Institute reported on the effect of aviation conditions on dental pulp and periostium (Project X91). In their preliminary work, 115 fillings of va ious types were inserted into uniform cavities prepared in extracted human teeth which were then placed in the pressure chamber at altitudes of 60,000 feet for twenty periods of one hour each. They found no evidence of displacement of the fillings following these exposures but felt that possibly during rapid changes of altitude oral fluids might be forced under leaking fillings and might account for toothaches experienced by flying personnel. In June, 1944, they reported that exposure of rats to altitudes of 24,000 to 26,000 feet for 25 three-hour periods did not affect the rate of growth of the incisor teeth but did disturb the calcification of dentin. No histological changes appeared in teeth so exposed.

Brickman and Bierman studied, in the low pressure chamber (Project X157), the relationship of dental malocclusion to ear block. In March, 1943, they reported that, of 447 subjects possessing normal occlusion, 5.8% developed ear block. Of 374 cases showing some degree of malocclusion, 23.7% developed ear block. Over-bite, retrusion, and protrusion were the chief offenders among the types of malocclusion. Of the methods for clearing ear block, movement of the mandible proved to be the most effective.

Bunch and Beaton at the Naval Air Station, Jacksonville, reported in March, 1945 on dental reaction to high altitude environment, (Project X355). They concluded that mechanical pressure from expansion of air trapped under fillings was not a usual cause of dental pain occurring at high altitudes. They felt that the pain in some way was a physiological phenomenon resulting from changes in barometric pressure associated with sudden variations of altitude, working on a mechanical basis.

Hutchins, Reynolds, Werner and Philbrook made an extensive study of aerodontalgia at the Marine Corps Air Station, Quantico, (Project X587). In July, 1945, they concluded that the pain of aerodontalgia is so severe in a large percentage of cases that the individual is distracted from performing important tasks; hence, aerodontalgia is of importance as a negative factor in successful aviation operations. They theorized that the majority of cases of dental pain occurring with altitude changes result from referred pain from the maxillary sinus and can be relieved by techniques similar to those used for relieving aero-otitis media. Since there is a tendency for pain referred from the maxillary sinus to localize in teeth with abnormalities, it is considered essential that good oral hygiene and regular dental examinations be recommended for all aviation personnel.

In Project X604, the Naval Medical Research Institute and the Naval Dental School are working on an evaluation of the low pressure chamber as a diagnostic aid in dentistry.

D. EAR, NOSE AND THROAT

General Survey

The chief ear, nose and throat problems in aviation to date have been those of aero-otitis media and aero-sinusitis in acute conditions and deafness as a chronic disturbance. Extensive work has been done at various aviation medical activities to support the conclusion that effective maintenance of nasal ventilation is highly desirable to enable Eustachian tube equalization. Techniques have been evolved to re-inflate the middle ear after descent from high altitude in cases where the subject has been unable to accomplish this voluntarily. The use of nasal constrictors as an adjuvant to these techniques has been recommended. Nose clips to aid dive-bombing pilots in equalizing middle ear pressures have been suggested and partially evaluated at ComFair, Quonset. (Project X685). Experienced pilots tend to reject these clips because of the necessity for applying them just before the dive and of removing the oxygen mask in order to accomplish this. However, inexperienced pilots who have formed no prejudiced conclusions about their equipment tend to accept these clips more readily. Work on this problem is continuing in the early stages of flight training.

Loss of hearing that occurs frequently in aviation personnel has been attacked by various ear "defenders" and "wardens". One of these, the V-51R ear warden, was officially adopted by the Navy.

E. FOOD AND WATER

Food

Special problems regarding the feeding of flight personnel were studied in naval laboratories and in civilian laboratories at the suggestion of the Navy. The most important contribution in aviation medical research in this field was the provision of emergency rations to be carried in the aviator's personal gear. As a result of laboratory and field tests conducted by the Naval Medical Research Institute, a candy ration was adopted for general use by the Bureau of Aeronautics. This replaced such items as pemmican and high protein food which were found to increase dehydration because of the necessity for excreting large quantities of water for dilution of the nitrogen metabolites. The candy ration is reasonably satisfactory for tropical areas but has certain disadvantages under cold weather cond tions. This investigation is still underway.

The Navy did not carry out much work in its own laboratories on the effects of diet on altitude tolerance. However, active liaison was maintained with laboratories at the University of Chicago and Columbia University where results of studies showed definite advantages of a high carbohydrate meal on subsequent altitude tolerance. The Navy's own program was directed chiefly toward the development of more adequate in-flight feeding, such as the provision of hot food to replace chocolate bars and crackers. During the latter part of the war, certain naval air transport planes were equipped with apparatus for preparation of complete meals from frozen "sky plates" prepared by the Maxson Food System. Messes at air stations for transient flyers were somewhat inadequate and became the subject of study by flight surgeons.

Representatives from naval aviation medical activities actively participated in various field trials of emergency rations carried out by the Army Air Forces and other agencies. An active part was also taken in the operations of the Air-Sea Rescue Agency.

Efforts were directed toward the establishment of minimum standards for quantity and quality of food as well as toward the more intimate details of the composition of rations. Problems encountered in aviation were unique in that compactness and weight were of primary importance.

Water

In aviation, the problem of supplying emergency drinking water was made more critical by limited storage space and stringent weight requirements. The application of zeolites for the desalination of sea water was brought about by cooperative efforts of the Naval Medical Research Institute and the Permutit Company. On the basis of a great many laboratory and field investigations, a satisfactory desalination kit was prepared and adopted for service use by the Bureau of Aeronautics. This was introduced into the Bureau of Aeronautics emergency life rafts and to some extent replaced canned water in seat packs. Final evaluation of the relative advantages and disadvantages of the desalination kit and canned water has yet to be made.

As a corollary to the development of the desalination kit, investigations were conducted on the physiological action of the salts remaining in sea water after use of the kit, a survey of bacteria in sea water, and the establishment of sta dards for emergency drinking water supplies.

While the Navy did not play a large part in developing solar stills, most naval activities concerned with air-sea rescue problems carried out tests on solar stills for comparison with other sources of drinking water. A very active liaison was maintained with the Personal Equipment Laboratory, Army Air Forces, Wright Field, and the Air-Sea Rescue Agency.

In connection with emergency drinking water and emergency food supplies, Medical Department personnel, in cooperation with civilian laboratories, were active in the establishment of minimal requirements for rations and water, as well as in the preparation of numerous manuals on survival promulgated by the Bureau of Supplies and Accounts, the Bureau of Naval Personnel, Chief of Naval Operations, Air-Sea Rescue Agency, and the Army Air Forces.

F. MOTION SICKNESS

Specific Projects

Lilienthal, at Pensacola, in Projects X72 and X252 found an incidence of air sickness of approximately 13% among aviation cadets; in rough air this rose to 30%, while, if rough air were avoided, it was as low as 6.5%. Hyoscine hydrobromide, in doses of 0.6 mgm. given 30 to 60 minutes before a flight, was reported to be a powerful preventive of air sickness and to have no undesirable side effects. There is no evidence that hyoscine delays or prevents adaptation to motion in flight. In fact, its efficacy suggests that it facilitates rapid adaptation to motion in flight.

Birren, Stormont, and Fisher at the Naval Medical Research Institute conducted an extensive investigation into motion sickness in Project X278 which is still continuing. They found no undesirable side effects to hyoscine-containing formulae but reported distinct undesirable effects to bulbocapnine; this latter drug had no effect as a depressant on motion sickness. Using a questionnaire technique, they found no evidence to indicate a correlation between general psychomatic complaints and susceptibility to sea sickness, although they considered that such a questionnaire might be useful in screening out persons who would be severely affected by sea sickness. Susceptible and non-susceptible subjects were tested on a rolling platform, simulating motion resulting from the rolling and pitching of a ship.

G. NITROGEN

Specific Projects

In 1942, workers at the Experimental Diving Unit, Navy Yard, Washinton, D. C. measured gaseous exchange under conditions simulating aviation and deep sea diving. The procedure of inhalation of radioactive krypton was followed in order to determine whether or not the rate of saturation of the tissues in the lower forearm and hand could be employed as an index of susceptibility to decompression sickness. (Project X43). They found that this test could not be used to determine specific susceptibility to aero-embolism but that the technique gave a precise basic physiological estimation which, under better quantitative control, might be used to estimate physical fitness.

In 1943, these same workers determined that exercise with pre-oxygenation substantially reduces the time required for decompression. They also confirmed previous studies showing that susceptibility to "bends" is apparently influenced by alcohol, disease, increasing age, and previous attacks of decompression sickness.

Gemmill reported from Pensacola in February, 1943 on the effect of pre-oxygenation on aero-embolism (Project X441) and concluded that, following one hour of pre-oxygenation at rest at sea level, 88% of susceptible individuals were protected from incapacitating symptoms of decompression sickness at 35,000 feet for four hours. McGoldrick, Lally and Langley in November, 1943, reported on the influence of demand and diluter demand oxygen systems used from sea level on the incidence of "bends" (Project X201). In the group studied, the percentage of "bends" of any degree was significantly greater in subjects using diluter demand equipment but there was no significant difference in the percentage of incapacitating "bends" between the group breathing 100% oxygen and the group using the diluter demand equipment.

In Project X284, Naval Medical Research Institute workers studied the effects of decompression on the specific gravity of specific tissues. In March, 1944, they reported on the observation of extravascular gas bubbles in tissues rich in fat, in adrenal cortex, and in nerve fibers but not in liver, skeletal muscle and tendon. Intravascular gas bubbles occurred in all these tissues but were far more numerous in those rich in fat. A significant fall was observed in the specific gravity of the entire animal after decompression, this decrease being greater in fat animals than in lean ones. The specific gravity of specific tissues was found to be inversely related to the total fat content and directly related to the water content of the given tissues.

In January, 1944, Welham, Blanch and Behnke at the Naval Medical Research Institute suggested a test for selection of personnel resistant to decompression (Project X338). In this test, given in the low pressure chamber, the first procedure is to have the subjects undergo a period of one hour of rest and one hour of exercise at 38,000 feet to eliminate those most susceptible. The second stage consists of two hours of exercise at 38,000 feet; the most resistant men will develop no symptoms during this stage.

Smedal and Brown at Pensacola reported in September, 1945, on the incidence of "bends" pain in a short exposure to simulated altitudes of 26,000, 28,000, and 30,000 feet. (Project X609). They concluded that exercise markedly increased the incidence of "bends" and that a greater incidence of "bends" was encountered at higher temperatures than at lower temperatures. At low altitudes (30,000 feet and below) with exposure of 20 minutes, the incidence of "bends" in resting subjects is very low and no temperature effect is apparent.

H. ORIENTATION IN FLIGHT

Specific Projects

Project X148

This general subject, Orientation in Flight, is being thoroughly investigated by Graybiel and co-workers at Pensacola who have already compiled an extensive series of reports on their findings.

Autokinesis

In September, 1944, tests were conducted on the effect of various arrangements of aircraft lights in reducing autokinesis. It was found that lights should be so arranged that at least three similar lights, as widely separated as possible, are visible from any angle. In addition to reducing the incidence of autokinesis, this arrangement is advantageous in giving depth perception clues.

In February, 1945, Graybiel, et al, reported on the autokinetic illusion and its significance in night flying. They found the illusion to be universally experienced by normal persons, who frequently, even under relatively simple laboratory conditions, cannot distinguish real from apparent motion. They described the phenomenon minutely and discussed the factors which tend to increase and decrease the frequency of appearance of the illusion. They recommended that aviators and probably the operators of certain other means of transportation be taught the characteristics of the phenomenon and the practical means by which it may be reduced.

Oculo-Gyral Illusion

In November, 1945, this group reported on the oculo-gyral illusion changes which may be observed following stimulation of the semicircular canals. They found the illusion to be more easily produced in dim than in bright illumination, to be unaffected by the administration of hyoscine hydrobromide in relatively large doses, and to provide a simple means of studying the sensitivity of the receptors in the semicircular canals. They considered the illusion to be of considerable importance in night flying.

Other Work

In March, 1946, this group reported on a new device for checiing the illusory perception of movement caused by angular acceleration and by centrifugal force during flight. This device with which observations are made in complete darkness during various flying maneuvers, consists of a collimated "star" installed in the rear cockpit of a training plane, the observer's and pilot's reports being recorded during flight. They found that forces engendered by various flight maneuvers are sufficient to produce marked illusory perceptions of movement and displacement of an objectively motionless object observed in the dark. The assumption is warranted that these illusions probably have contributed to disorientation and accidents in night flying.

Additional studies using new devices for measureing angular acceleration and "g" in three components, with recording of these factors simultaneously with the observer's verbal reports, will be carried out as this project continues.

Project X259

Beals and Luykx, working at the Naval Air Station, Anacostia, conducted a study under Project X259 on disorientation of pilots in night and instrument flying. They found that 1400 hours of flight experience gave the dividing line between "spinners" and "non-spinners". They felt that this degree of experience brought about sufficient familiarity with disorientation problems that these could be solved in flight. They recommended increased instruction in the hazards of disorientation during flight training.

I. OXYGEN

1. Anoxia, Demonstration of

Specific Projects

In Project X10, Gemmill reported on the development of standard procedures for the measurement of altitude tolerance. He concluded that the dotter apparatus is useful in obtaining a quantitative distinction in a man's performance between normal and severe anoxia but is unsatisfactory for moderate degrees of anoxia. No deviation from the base line results were obtained at simulated altitudes of 8,000 to 12,000 feet but marked changes were found at 18,000 feet. The Wickes' psychomotor apparatus was found to require too long a training period to enable it to be easily employed in routine testing and it was found to give an inadequate index of anoxia at 18,000 feet. The flicker fusion apparatus was found to be valuable for experimental purposes, but to require too much training to make it practical for mass testing. This last conclusion was concurred in by Ivy working at the Naval Medical Research Institute, (Project X32).

In Project X111, direct comparison of flicker fusion and dotter tests under comparative conditions of anoxia was made. It was finally concluded that neither of these tests could be recommended for selection of an individual with respect to his response to anoxia.

Hecht and Peckham, working at Pensacola, reported in March, 1943, on the influence of anoxia on contrast discrimination, (Project X153). They first conducted tests on 16 subjects, all of whom, without oxygen, showed significant deterioration in contrast discrimination. On a second trial, 57% of subjects showed loss of contrast discrimination, 13% showed no loss, 16% showed gain, while 14% performed the test incorrectly. They concluded that the contrast discrimination test which they used was unsatisfactory because of the failure of large portions of the population to show anoxic effects.

In December, 1943, Draeger and Fauley at the Naval Medical Research Institute, (Project X159), attempted to develop a simplified electronic fusion flicker apparatus for use in flight to detect anoxia before it became severe enough to impair judgment. They concluded that the determination of the flicker fusion threshold cannot be recommended as a means of detecting anoxia in aircraft crews while in flight because of the time required for partial dark adaptation, variations existing among individuals, and the need for someone to operate the equipment.

Gerstell at the Naval Air Station, Seattle, developed a card-sorting test to demonstrate the effects of anoxia in the low pressure chamber,

(Project X282). In this test, 89% of 200 individuals scored better at 30,000 feet with oxygen than at 18,000 feet without oxygen. In Project X283, West, Brown, James and Burt at Pensacola, concluded that this card-sorting test was unsuitable for use because learning greatly influenced the test results, because the results under anoxia were influenced by compensating factors, and because the test was relatively difficult and bulky for use in pressure chambers.

Brown in October, 1944, reported from Pensacola on Project X431, (development of anoxia demonstration procedure for altitude training units on basis of breath-holding ability). His iirst report stated that 208 of 212 subjects showed a marked decrease in breath-holding ability at 18,000 feet without oxygen as compared to that at sea level. He felt that this reduction in breath-holding ability at altitude was consistent enough to warrant investigation of its usefulness as a demonstration of the impaired function resulting from anoxia at altitude. In his second report, after further study of thss problem he concluded that the breath-holding procedure was less effective than mask-removal and slightly more effective than the letter cancellation test in convincing personnel of the necessity for the use of oxygen at high altitude.

In September, 1945, Moore, Nuzie and Sonn of the Naval Air Station, Vero Beach, Florida, (Project X564), reported on the development of a new "M-N" device for demonstrating anoxic effects on night and day vision. This apparatus consisted of monocular and binocular "scopes" constructed to allow the observer to view slides of aircraft silhouettes under illumination approximating starlight and also average daylight. They concluded that 90 to 96% of subjects tested in a low pressure chamber were convinced subjectively and objectively that anoxia impaired night vision. Ninety-eight percent of those tests were also convinced objectively of the anoxic effect on macular vision. This group recommended the adoption of this device for all altitude training units and for use as a test of night visual acuity.

In Project X580, Grinsted at ComFair, Quonset, reported the development of a new device for low pressure chamber demonstration of the effect of anoxia on night vision. This was found to be very effective, 100% of subjects noting the effect of anoxia on night vision in the darkened chamber at a simulated altitude of 10,000 feet. Grinsted's apparatus was improved at the Naval Air Station, Grosse, Ile, Michigan, by making it smaller and more adaptable for chamber use. In Project X667, Smedal, Hoffman, Brown and Dougherty, working at the Naval Air Station, Pensacola, evaluated the Grinsted device. They concluded that 93% of subjects were aware of improvement in their vision when given 100% oxygen, in comparison with the anoxic level of vision when exposed to 12,000 feet. They thus confirmed the original conclusions of the Quonset Group.

Seitz at the Altitude Training Unit, Naval Air Station, Miami, reported in Project X593 on the measurement and demonstration of loss of visual function associated with anoxia. He concluded: (1) loss in range for targets observed under conditions of low illumination is evident at 5,000 feet; (2) the loss in range above 10,000 feet when supplementary oxygen is not used is considerable; (3) the effect of anoxia on vision at altitudes below 10,000 feet is small and not considered of operational significance. Hence, supplementary oxygen was considered unnecessary below 12,000 feet. These results were questioned by the oxygen training unit under the Division of Aviation Medicine, Bureau of Medicine and Surgery and a project to investigate this problem further has been suggested.

Price and Fuller at the Naval Air Station, Alameda, California, investigated the effect of altitudes of 10,000 feet and 12,000 feet on form perception at low levels of illumination using the Radium Plaque Adaptometer,(Project X538). They concluded that there were no statistically reliable differences among altitudes of sea level, 10,000 feet and 12,000 feet. These experiments suggest that form perception of the completely dark adapted eye is not affected by the reduced barometric pressure of a simulated altitude of 10,000 feet. Hence, this work and that of Seitz, mentioned above, are in agreement, but the methods utilized are considered by many to be open to question.

While the work outlined above leaves somewhat unsettled the best methods for demonstrating and/or measuring the effects of mild anoxia, experience in both service and civilian laboratories leaves little doubt that exposures to altitudes above 10,000 feet without oxygen present distinct physiological problems to the body. The chief difficulty in all measurements is that the degree to which the body has compensated for the additional load is not included in the test procedure. Thus, compensations may be made without appreciable objective or subjective signs, yet the situation may be physiologically very different from that at sea level. It is considered that one of the most important fundamental problems remaining in the evaluation of all types of equipment and measures for high altitude work is the development of better methods for assaying the true physiological state of the individual.

2. Oxygen Equipment

Development of Navy Oxygen Equipment

Early in the war, the most pressing problems were those of oxygen supply. The procurement of some type of oxygen equipment, suitable for long flights in the old Catalina patrol planes was extremely urgent, and the question of oxygen economy was paramount. Partly for these reasons, a rebreather type system, using an oxygen regenerating chemical for both CO_2 absorption and supplementary oxygen production, was adopted.

One of the important problems of that time was the balancing of obvious physiological disadvantages of the rebreather type apparatus against the gains accruing from its oxygen economy. The Engineering Division, Bureau of Aeronautics, established a contract with the National Institute of Health, U. S. Public Health Service, to evaluate exactly what the rebreather could and could not do. This was essential since this device was already in service in large numbers. Meanwhile, a group at the Experimental Diving Unit demonstrated the FWB recirculator which had certain advantages, as well as certain disadvantages as compared with the Navy rebreather. The Medical Research Section, along with the Division of Aviation Medicine, Bureau of Medicine and Surgery, sponsored experimental work leading to a more adequate comparison of these two devices, and concluded that, in spite of its greater comfort, the lack of a demand feature in the FWB recirculator prevented its general adoption.

During the period discussed, many Navy fighter planes were equipped with a demand-type apparatus which, while having certain features superior to the rebreather, required large supplies of oxygen. Under the sponsorship of the Army Air Forces, various manufacturers were modifying the demand apparatus by incorporation of a diluter valve which would admit measured quantities of ambient air at altitudes below 30,000 feet. This type of apparatus offered many advantages over the rebreather type, but still required considerably more compressed oxygen than the latter.

Meanwhile, the Subcommittee on Oxygen and Anoxia of the Committee on Aviation Medicine, National Research Council, had been formed. The Medical Research Section requested the aid of this group in the evaluation of Navy oxygen equipment and, through the equipment and Materials Branch, Bureau of Aeronautics, contracts were let with certain civilian laboratories and the Office of Scientific Research and Development for work on (a) improving the rebreather, and (b) evaluating the rebreather against diluter demand type equipment. At about this same time, the Naval Medical Research Institute was commissioned and certain phases of the oxygen problem were assigned to it.

The results of these several contracts indicated that the rebreather could be improved considerably; for example, by the use of "KOX" chemical rather than "GOX" chemical, the apparatus could be made extremely economical of cylinder oxygen, and by the use of automatic venting devices, somewhat safer. These additions increased both the cost and the complexity of the rebreather. For these reasons, and because of the simplicity and availability of the diluter demand type apparatus, the rebreather was finally discarded in favor of diluter demand regulator.

The final steps in coordinating the Navy oxygen program with that of the Army, (that is, adoption of diluter demand equipment), was accomplished after establishemnt of medical liaison in the Military Requirements Division, Bureau of Aeronautics and after the Medical Research Section, Bureau of Aeronautics had been transferred to the Bureau of Medicine and Surgery as the Aviation Branch of the Research Division of the last-mentioned bureau.

Oxygen Equipment for Therapeutic Purposes

As a result of the great volume of developmental work on aviation breathing equipment, medical personnel concerned therewith were called upon to aid in the design and evaluation of therapeutic oxygen equipment. Two main types of devices were developed namely, (1) continuous flow inhalators and (2) positive pressure resuscitators.

In connection with continuous flow systems, the Army type A8B (BLB) mask and A-11 regulator were modified for casualty evaluation installations. Also, with the aid of the Bureuu of Aeronautics, several modifications of systems designed for transpost aircraft were made available for use on casualty-evacuating LST's, Hospital Ships and so forth. The Bureau of Aeronautics provided to medical personnel many items of obsolete aircraft equipment which could be used for therapeutic purposes.

The development of resuscitators was greatly simulated by the serious toxic gas problems arising in connection with shipboard fires. In this development, the experience of personnel concerned with the aviation oxygen program was utilized for the evaluation of currently available resuscitation equipment. In the summer of 1945, for the first time, a resuscitator was placed on the Bureau of Medicine and Surgery supply table.

In considering problems of the administration of therapeutic oxygen, it was apparent that methods for applying artificial respiration were in need of thorough re-evaluation. In liaison with the Council on Physical Medicine of the American Medical Association, the National Research Council and the Army, such an evaluation was undertaken. As a part of this work, the Research Division, in cooperation with the Division of Medical Statistics, Bureau of Medicine and Surgery, prepared a form letter which was forwarded to all ships and stations for reporting cases of asphyxia requiring artificial respiration.

Aviation Medical Activities cooperated with BuShips and other agencies in attempts to provide more adequate protection against smoke from shipboard fires. Instances such as the holocasst aboard the carrier, USS FRANKLIN, greatly stimulated the interest of aviation medical personnel in this problem. Just before the cessation of hostilities, several devices, based on modification of aircraft oxygen equipment, had been studied at the Naval Medical Research Institute, the Naval Research Laboratory and the National Institute of Health. These devices would very probably have aided operational use had the need therefor continued.

Development of Oxygen Masks

During the course of the war, various naval activities tested a large number of oxygen masks, including one developed by the Aviation Branch Research Division, and termed the MRS-I mask. In general, the earlier efforts aimed toward devising masks which would fit perfectly, not freeze up at temperatures down to -65°F., be comfortable to wear for long periods, and be durable under service conditions. During the course of the testing program, it became obvious that some compromise with these factors would have to be tolerated. The Type A-14 mask, developed by the Mayo Clinic and the Army Air Forces, and manufactured by the Ohio Chemical Company, was finally adopted as standard for use with the diluter demand regulator. While a great deal of energy was expended upon the development of masks and improvements in suspension, it is difficult to outline any new principles which were found. For this reason, further discussion is limited to a listing of the various projects in the appendix.

OXYGEN

3. Oxygen Mask Leak Testing

General Survey-

One important development in c nnection with the testing of masks should be mentioned. This was the devising of suitable methods for determining oxygen mask leakage. In the early phases, tests such as presenting volatile substances in the region of the mask, were tried but these were unsatisfactory due to the fact that they failed to distinguish between significant and minor (and almost inevitable) amounts of leakage. Development of quantitative methods took two directions: (1) the so-called "spot" tests whi h were either gasometric or volumetric, and (2) analysis of expired air collected over a period of several minutes. After considerable controversy, the Bureau of Medicine and Surgery finally recommended to the Bureau of Aeronautics that simple "spot" tests using devices such as the McKesson Spirometer, be used for quick determinations of the adequacy of fit of a given airman's service mask; but that these be supplemented by the more time consuming methods involving collection of expired air and analysis thereof when it is desired to evaluate the fit of experimental masks or mask suspensions under consideration for service adoption.

Specific Projects

Gemmill reported from Pensacola in April, 1944, on a comparison of oxygen mask leak testing methods, (Project X288). He summarized leak testing methods under two types: (1) chemical and (2) mechanical. The two chemical methods now in use are the Scholander nitrogen analysis of mask air and the odor test. The mechanical testers depend on suction pressure for revealing the leak. He found that all of the mechanical testers gave a large number of false failures, chiefly because subjects find it difficult to hold their breath for the required 10 seconds, and also because movement of the subject's head or jaws frequently destroys the pressure relationship between the mask and the tester regardless of the fitting of the mask to the face. He finally concluded that the Scholander apparatus is the best tester for service use.

In a second report on this same project, Lilienthal, Riley and Fugitt worked on the conditions under which expired air may be used for mask fit testings. They compared nitrogen concentrations in inspired and expired air under controlled conditions, using the Scholander analysis test for evaluation of fit and comparing this with similar measurements made by the McKesson mask fit tests. They concluded: (1) after breathing of a constant high-oxygen, low-nitrogen mixture for 5 minutes, inspired and expired air samples are equivalent with respect to their nitrogen concentrations; (2) the nitrogen concentration of the collected expired air represents, in the presence of a mask leak, an average of the variable nitrogen concentrations inspired during the collection period. Therefore, the nitrogen concentration of collected expired air is a physiological significant index of mask fit. It is considered to be the best available standard of reference for other mask fits. The Scholander test performed on an inspiratory mask sample showed poor correlation with the nitrogen concentration of the collected expired air, whereas the same tests performed on an expiratory sample showed a much better correlation. The McKesson test occasionally yielded grossly inaccurate measurements of "normally" occurring leaks.

Henson, King, and Goldman, at the Naval Medical Research Institute, reported in April, 1944, on an evaluation of the McKesson leak testing method for oxygen masks, (Project X312). They concluded that the Scholander technique is unreliable since the sample of mask air withdrawn for analysis may not be a representative one, chiefly because of inadequate mixing. They felt that a volumetric technique, such as the McKesson, is the method of choice for determining leakage, since it measures total leakage and does not depend upon the site of sampling. They suggested limits of leakage for specifications for acceptance of types of oxygen masks.

In May, 1944, Riley and Fugitt at Pensacola reported on a comparison of oxygen mask leak testing without special apparatus and by the Scholander nitrogen analyzer, (Project X389). They concluded that while many inexperienced subjects are unable to detect significant leaks by the inspiratory mask fit test, this test can be made adequately sensitive by refinements in technique, and is not affected adversely by conditions likely to obtain during high altitude flight. Almost all subjects, even though inexperienced, can detect significant leaks by the expiratory mask fit test under normal indoor conditions, but this test is adversely affected by conditions likely to obtain during high altitude flight.

In August, 1944, Fugitt reported in Project X422, on an evaluation of the McKesson pocket mask leak tester. He concluded that the accuracy of this tester is of the same order as the expiratory mask leak test without the aid of any special device. While it is not indispensable, it is as accurate as any other mechanical leak tester and could be used by those preferring such a method. It was considered to be unsuitable for issue as a personal issue item because of its bulk and the difficulty which untrained personnel experienced in using it. In Project X499, Fugitt evaluated a pocket mask leak tester made by the Master Plastics Molding Corporation and concluded that, because of its unreliability, and because simpler tests requiring no special devices seem superior, it was not suitable for service use. The group at the Naval Air Station,

San Diego, evaluated this latter leak tester in Project X477, and considered it to give results as reliable as those obtained by the Scholander method and to have certain advantages over the McKesson method.

Becuase the Pensacola and Naval Medical Research Institute workers did not agree on the best means of measuring the mask leaks, a conference was held to reconcile their differences and, in October, 1944, recommendations for changes in speci ications for oxygen mask leakage were proposed.

In Project X521, Fugitt at Pensacola studied the manner in which mask leaks change with varying negative pressures. He found that most mask leaks improve in fitting with added suction while some others become worse. He determined that the pressure, 2.0 centimeters of water, would serve as a satisfactory practical standard for mechanical leak testers.

In May, 1945, Fugitt reported further on tests of the McKesson Spirometer type tester (Project X565), and concluded that mechanical leak testers of the McKesson type are suitable only in a quantitative sense and are unsatisfactory as a means of accurately measuring the size of the mask leak.

The Royal Canadian Air Force oxygen mask leak tester was evaluated in September, 1945, by Weatherby at Pensacola, (Project X665). He concluded that its greater complexity of design, operation and maintenance, as compared to collapsible testers, (as advocated by the Bureau of Aeronautics) made it undesirable for Navy use.

In March, 1946, Skow and Vaughan at Pensacoaa reported on a modified McKesson pocket oxygen mask leak tester, (Project X698). They found that this tester was greatly improved over earlier models, with an excellent low loading of 1.4 centimeters. The addition of a breathing vent enables more accurate tests by decreasing the necessary breath-holding time, making possible several tests in the time required previously for one test and also lessening the physiological and physical disturbance caused the subject. They considered it superior to the standard Scholander technique and to the previously available pocket-type volumetric equipment.

OXYGEN

4. Liquid and Chemical Oxygen

Chemical Oxygen

On the basis of convenience and economy of weight, it was considered desirable to carry oxygen for breathing purposes in the form of a stable, chemical compound which could be made to liberate gaseous oxygen when desired. Chemicals as a source of oxygen for use in aviation were first utilized in the Navy rebreather. A substance known as "GOX", a mixture of alkaline peroxides, mainly sodium peroxide, served both to absorb CO_2 and to produce from 1/3 to 1/2 of the total oxygen supplied during a run.

For a number of years, the Naval Research Laboratory engaged in experimental work on the development of peroxides of metals other than sodium and in cooperation with the DuPont Company developed a material known as "KOX". This consisted chiefly of potassium tetroxide and supplied a much larger amount of oxygen than the earlier chemical. In fact, during most of its useful life, a suitable canister filled with this material produces oxygen in excess of the user's demand, which excess can be employed for flushing nitrogen from the rebreather system. Physiological developmental work on this material was carried out at the National Institute of Health, U. S. Public Health Service under a contract with the Bureau of Aeronautics, with supplementary investigations at the Naval Medical Research Institute and Pensacola. This material was utilized in a rebreather system having obvious disadvantages and therefore was not used operationally to any great extent, although pilot batches were produced by the Mine Safety Appliances Company.

In the early part of the war, the British utilized an "oxygen candle" for supplying oxygen in small submarines. This device was adapted to aviation use through the cooperative efforts of the Naval Research Laboratory, the University of Pennsylvania, the National Defense Research Committee and the Mine Safety Appliances Company under contract with the Bureau of Aeronautics. In one form, it was incorporated in the apparatus with a continuous flow of approximately 20 minutes' duration; in another form, it was combined with the "KOX" described above in a 2-hour rebreather apparatus, designated the "C-K" unit. Both of these developments were actually consummated in civilian laboratories but the basic research was sponsored by the Navy. Neither unit was available in time for operational use during the war. Toxicological analyses of the gases from the oxygen candle were carried out at the Naval Medical Research Institute.

Liquid Oxygen

On a volume basis, liquid oxygen is the most economical form for transporting large quantities of oxygen for use in breathing equipment. During the war, numerous projects were conducted cooperatively by Bureau of Aeronautics and Bureau of Medicine and Surgery activities in an attempt to adapt this source to use in aircraft. Two types of apparatus were worked on most extensively. One, developed by Mathis and Milan, utilized electrical energy to convert the liquid to a gas. The other device, the Ackerman converter, utilized the temperature of the surroundings, which is always considerably above that of liquid oxygen, to effect the transformation. Physiological problems were not numerous, except those concerned with (a) the establishment of Peak rates of flow required from a converter designed for multi place aircraft and (b) the possible inhalation of oxygen at very low temperatures. These problems were investigated at Pensacola, and Patuxent, with the cooperation of engineers and physiologists of the Bureau of Aeronautics, the Bureau of Medicine and Surgery, the Naval Research Laboratory, the National Institute of Health, Naval Air Station, Anascostia and various civilian laboratories. Owing to a number of engineering difficulties, liquid oxygen was never installed in any considerable number of naval aircraft although many test runs were made and small quantities were transported to forward areas in special containers developed by the Bureau of Aeronautics and the Bureau of Ships.

Specific Projects

In Project X644, the group at Pensacola reported on tests of the Ackerman liquid oxygen converter and concluded that it was fundamentally sound in principle. However, peak flow characteristics of this device were not completely satisfactory and modifications were suggested. In this same project, the Dewar flask was reported on with the conclusion that it was unreliable for service use because of potential danger if collaspe fo the concentric spheres. In reporting on the Mathis-Milan converter, the Pensacola group concluded that, considering all aspects, this device was a practical unit for service use.

In Project X618, the group at Patuxent reported on problems dealing with the transportation and handling of liquid oxygen for aircraft use and suggested appropriate means for this handling.

In November, 1945, Catchpole and Rohrbach at the Naval Medical Research Institute reported on the evaluation of chemicals as a source of oxygen supply for aircraft use, (Project X586). They tested the chlorate candles devised by the Naval Research Laboratory and concluded that, while these candles gave percentages of oxygen ranging from 95.6% to 97.2% and insignificant amounts of CO and CO_2, the initial smoke was frequently unpleasant and sometimes irritating enough to necessitate removal of the mask. They further concluded that while no deleterious after-effects were observed as a result of breathing total gases from these candles, more effective filtration of the gases to remove the undesirable respiratory effects should be attempted. Work on this project is continuing.

OXYGEN

5. Low Pressure Chamber Indoctrination and Training

Specific Projects

In Project X38, the Pensacola Altitude Training Unit reported on the repeat reliability of classification runs in the low pressure chamber at 35,000 feet. It was concluded that a 1-hour run was not an absolute test for classification. Using four 1-hour runs on successive days and a 1-hour run followed by a 4-hour run on the following day, the majority of failures occurred in the 1-hour test and in the first three hours of the 4-hour test.

In November, 1945, the Altitude Training Unit at the Naval Air Station, Norfolk, evaluated the oxygen and altitude indoctrination program, (Project X501). On checking aviation personnel to determine their knowledge of oxygen equipment, it was found that the ability to use this equipment deteriorates very rapidly, especially when no repeated instructions are given periodically. Men who had had an introductory oxygen lecture, or who had become acquainted with the equipment longer than six months before this evaluation, had no better knowledge of the equipment than the men who had had no previous experience with it. In a second report, they concluded that, while lectures, low pressure chamber "flights" and actual aircraft flights are all valuable in contributing to knowledge of oxygen equipment, experience with actual oxygen equipment in aircraft is the most influential single factor. Personnel who obtained their experience in single engine carrier-based planes tended to know more about the use of oxygen than those associated with multi-engine land-based planes. Groups who had had oxygen experience in combat flying, however, did no better in a test involving knowledge of oxygen euuipment than those who had had non-combat oxygen experience. Although a flight in the low pressure chamber was beneficial for an initial indoctrination, flights beyond one did not add anything to the individual's knowledge of the use of oxygen, as measured by the Norfolk tests.

OXYGEN

6. Physiology

General Summary

While a large part of the time spent on altitude problems was necessarily directed toward the evaluation of specific items of equipment, it was possible, especially in the research laboratory at Pensacola, to carry out certain basic studies on the physiological changes occurring under conditions of anoxia. These studies are in addition to those on vision which are discussed separately.

The work at Pensacola was greatly aided by the development by Drs. Riley and Lilienthal of a method for the direct estimation of the gas tensions in blood samples obtained by skillful use of an indwelling arterial needle. Among these basic studies were, (a) findings showing that great variations may occur in the arterial oxygen tension in different individuals under conditions of exercise at altitude and (b) the development of a new method for the determination of effective alveolar gas tensions.

Another line of investigation, bearing directly on the physiology of anoxia, was the study of "emergency breathing techniques". These studies were conducted at Corpus Christi, Pensacola, Miami and the Naval Medical Research Institute. They are discussed in some detail in connection with pressure breathing.

Development of suitable tests for assaying the physiological state of an individual under conditions of anoxia, (exclusive of vision changes discussed elsewhere), was carried out at the Naval Medical Research Institute in collaboration with the National Research Council. A set of standard tests was proposed but these have not as yet been generally adopted.

This is an important field which warranted much more emphasis than it received during the war because the validity of any evaluation of specific items of equipment depends greatly upon the criteria employed. It is however, a difficult field, and results could not be obtained with the rapidity necessary to war problems. Work is being continued at the Naval Medical Research Institute.

Establishment of Physiological Criteria

In Septe ber, 1943, the Vice Chief of Naval Operations designated the Bureau of Medicine and Surgery as the agency for the establishment and promulgation of the physiological requirements for all oxygen breathing appliances, and for all other equipment involving physiological considerations, as a basis for the design of such equipment. While this letter was addressed to all Bureaus and Offices of the Navy Department, the most active research developed thereby was in the design of aviation equipment by the Bureau of Aeronautics. To make the task of the engineers easier, the Aviation Branch, Research Division, Bureau of Medicine and Surgery, prepared a set of physiological specifications for the design of oxygen equipment. These specifications were based on the best knowledge available at the time and were forwarded to the Bureau of Aeronautics by official letter dated 22 October 1943. This letter dealt with such items as desirable altitudes for wearing oxygen equipment, data for calculating the duration of oxygen supply, maximum tolerable resistances in oxygen breathing equipment, minimum concentrations of oxygen in the inspired air as a function of altitude, limiting pressure for pressure breathing equipment, etc.

In preparing these criteria, it became apparent that there existed serious gaps in physiological knowledge at certain points. Several research projects were established to obtain necessary information. In addition, the cooperation of the National Research Council, was requested. As a result of this request, the Subcommittee on Oxygen and Anoxia, under the Committee on Aviation Medicine produced a volume entitled "Handbook of Respiratory Data in Aviation".

In 1944, and 1945, several conferences between representatives of the Navy, Army and civilian laboratories were called to discuss specific phases of such problems as pressure breathing, respiratory physiology as applied to aviation, etc. In the latter part of 1945, the Aviation Branch, Research Division, Bureau of Medicine and Surgery, felt that sufficient new information has been accumulated to revise the physiological criteria and to add items concerning bail-out equipment, mask leakage, safety pressure regulators, etc. These were prepared in final form in January, 1946 and forwarded to the Chief, Bureau of Aeronautics on 31 January. At the present time, they remain as the official physiological specifications for the design of aviation oxygen equipment.

During the period within which the physiological data for oxygen equipment were being studied, numerous other physiological problems assumed great imporatnce. For some time each individual problem was handled as a separate entity through medical liaison in the Bureau of Aeronautics and the Research Division as well as the Division of Aviation Medicine, Bureau of Medicine and Surgery. With the development of still more advanced type combat aircraft, it was considered desirable to forward such data as could be compiled in the form of official criteria. This was done in the summer of 1945 and, in August, such data were forwarded officially to the Bureau of Aeronautics. Such items as the physiological aspects of cabin pressurization, emergency escape from high-speed aircraft, decompression sickness, explosive decompression, ventilation, maximum and minimum standards for temperature and humidity, problems of acceleration and "g", and the optical properties of the aircraft canopy were included. These data are utilized in establishing policy regarding military characteristics of new type aircraft, and are subject to constant revision.

It is emphasized that the development of these criteria was, and is, based upon the work of many persons in numerous laboratories throughout the country and required arbitrary decisions in the case of many controversial points. Responsibility for these decisions, right or wrong, rests with tee Aviaition Branch, Research Division, and the medical liaison officers to the Bureau of Aeronautics.

Specific Projects

Lilienthal and Riley at Pensacola, (Project X323), in February, 1944, adapted the micro-gasometric method of Roughton and Scholander to the determination of oxygen saturations of "capillary" blood. The oxygen saturations of "capillary" blood obtained from the heated earlobe were compared with samples of arterial blood obtained simultaneously from the brachial artery and found to correspond withing the limits of analytical accuracy, to the arterial oxygen saturations under a variety of conditions and levels of anoxemia. They concluded that this method furnishes a simple and accurate means of determining arterial oxygen saturations without recourse to arterial puncture.

In a second report under this project, they concluded that the Scholander nitrogen analyzer provides a simple rapid method for the determination of nitrogen in high-oxygen low-nitrogen gas mixtures. Calibrating each burette gives accuracy sufficient for a variety of physiological studies; by means of appropriate correction factors, the method may be used at various pressure altitudes up to 40,000 feet.

The Scholander-Roughton method for determining the CO_2 content of the blood was tested and the findings of Scholander and Roughton confirmed. In addition, the CO_2 contents of samples of blood drawn simultaneously from the brachial artery and from the heated earlobe were found to be equivalent.

In a final report on this project, the authors studied the arterial oxyhemoglobin saturations in men breathing various oxygen-nitrogen mixtures at critical pressure altitudes in the decompression chamber. These findings, consisting of 43 observations on 24 subjects at 20,000, 35,000, and 40,000 feet, established these realtionships: (a) the oxyhemoglobin saturation may be predicted with an accuracy of plus or minus 3% for a given oxygen-nitrogen mixture at these pressure altitudes; (b) the arterial oxyhemoglobin saturation may fall appreciably during a short period of medium to heavy work in states of mild anoxia, during which work, certain undetermined factors operate to make the saturation unpredictable.

In Project X484, Gemmill and Malone reported in May, 1945, on the relationship between alveolar air oxygen tensions and arterial blood oxygen saturations. They made determinations of oxygen tensions and oxygen blood saturations on men during rest and work at altitude. During rest, there was good agreement between alveolar air oxygen tension, as determined, and the arterial oxygen tension, (calculated from an oxygen hemoglobin dissociation curve and the determined blood saturation). During work at altitude, there was a spread between these two values. They concluded that, when the double stress of work and anoxia is placed on man, the arterial blood is no longer is equilibrium with alveolar air oxygen tensions, since the oxygen saturation of arterial blood falls. Therefore, the ability of the body to keep the arterial blood saturated at the same tension as the alveolar is limited. For this reason, a man working at altitude should be protected from these changes by the use of his oxygen equipment.

In January, 1946, Riley and Lilienthal, working on this same project, devised an indirect method for calculating alveolar gas pressures, which requires simply the determination of arterial pCO_2, and the pO_2 and the pCO_2 of inspired and expired air. Their theoretical analysis indicates that alveolar gas pressures so determined represent the physiologically effective mean pressures and are not subject to errors introduced by "time" and "space" factors. This indirect method avoids the difficulties inherent in the classical direct methods for sampling alveolar air, especially on subjects during exercise.

In a third report on the project, Lilienthal and Riley discussed the physiological implications of the oxygen pressure gradient from alveolar air to arterial boood during rest and exercise at sea level and at altitude.

The Pensacola group, in Project X475, is continuing work on the determination of aqueous vapor tension in expired air.

In May, 1945, Fugitt reported from Pensacola on his investigation of isothermy expansion of gases saturated with water vapor, (Project X579). He made experimental demonstration of the manner in which gases saturated with water vapor expand iso-thermally and he presented volumetric and gravometric data on this. He concluded that the theoretical calculation based upon Dalton's law of Partial Pressures accurately confirmed his observed data.

In January, 1945, Riley reported on a direct method for the determination of oxygen and carbon dioxide tensions in blood (Project X450).

This method involves the equilibration of a bubble of gas with blood at 37 °C. and the analysis of this bubble for CO_2 and O_2. The Roughton-Scholander syringe is used both as an equilibration chamber and a bubble analyzer, thus eliminating any transfer of the bubble. Comparing the results of this technique with those obtained using a tonometer at sea level, they agreed very closely for both CO_2 and O_2. Comparing the results at altitude in the low pressure chamber, the method was also found accurate enough for practical purposes. Riley, concluded that this technique is sufficiently simple, quick, and accurate for practical application to problems in respiratory physiology.

In a second report in July, 1945, Riley described modifications in his original method to increase its accuracy. He concluded that a significant improvement in the accuracy of CO_2 tension determinations had been achieved and that the upper limit of the range in which oxygen tensions could be determined with useful accuracy had been extended to at least 100 mm.Hg.

Weatherby and Burt in July, 1944, reported on Project X402 from Pensacola. They studied the individual variation in respiratory responses to CO_2 at altitude and concluded that this response of a group of subjects to CO_2 was the same at 15,000 feet pressure altitude as at sea level when the same tension of CO_2 in the inspired air was used in both cases. Therefore, the respiratory response to CO_2 at this altitude is not altered by anoxia.

The altitude training unit at the Naval Air Station, Miami reported in January, 1944, on the effect of temperature on anoxic failure in altitude chambers, (Project X396). It had been noted that the average incidence for failure at 18,000 feet approximated 3.0% in ordinary low pressure chamber runs, whereas only 0.3% of men given chilled runs showed anoxic failure at this altitude. It was shown that the accumulation of oxygen was no different in the warm or cold runs. They suggested that improved vascular tone, due to cold and shivering, increases resistance to vaso-motor collapse, despite the increase in oxygen consumption due to the cold and shivering.

Pecora and Consolazio at the Naval Medical Research Institute in December, 1944, checked the reliability of the technique suggested by Lilienthal and Riley for the determination of arterial oxygen saturation from samples of capillary blood, (Project X373). They concluded that the method was accurate for experimentation but should be limited to use by experienced personnel possessing a background in gas analysis, because considerable practice is necessary even for experienced personnel to obtain reliable data.

Farr at the Naval Medical Research Institute in Project X250, studied the urea clearance of men exposed to simulated altitudes of 18,000 feet for one hour in a low pressure chamber and found that this exposure did not significantly change the clearance.

Ivy and Behnke from the Naval Medical Research Institute, (Project X116), in February, 1943, reported on pressure breathing physiology, and pressure breathing equipment. Using the "pneumolotar" of the General Electric X-ray Corporation, subjects were enabled to undergo flights to 45,000 and 50,000 feet in the low pressure chamber without any other equipment. Intermittent pressure breathing of air enables individuals to remain at 22,000 feet for 30 minutes without distress and at 25,000 feet for 15 minutes with some distress, when the pressure is of the order of eight inches H_2O. This increase in "ceiling" of about 6,000 feet should greatly increase the safety of oxygen administration for the aviator.

A study of oxygen and carbon dioxide dissociation curves in vivo under normal conditions and during anoxia and acapnia was made in September, 1945, by Riley and Lilienthal in Project X490. They concluded that standard oxyhemoglobin dissociation curves accurately describe conditions as they exist in vivo under a variety of physiological states of rest and stress.

Hoffman, Clark and Brown from the Altitude Training Unit at Pensacola conducted studies on the rates of fall of blood oxygen saturation at simulated altitudes following mask removals, (Project X572). At altitudes of 28,000 feet and above, a subject's mask was removed; he then performed a simple card sorting task while his reactions were noted and recorded. When unconsciousness was imminent, the mask was replaced and 100% oxygen administered; blood oxygen saturations were estimated throughout the procedure with a Millikan oximeter while ambient oxygen pressure was determined with a continuous oxygen analyzer. This procedure was repeated on 25 individuals at each of four altitudes: 28,000, 30,000, 35,000 and 38,000 feet. They found that average times to imminent unconsciousness were 141 seconds at 28,000 feet, 98 seconds at 30,000 feet, 72 seconds at 35,000 feet and 47 seconds at 38,000 feet, while average times of useful consciousness as determined by the appearance of the first error in card sorting were 110 seconds at 28,000 feet, 73 seconds at 30,000 feet, 46 seconds at 35,000 feet, and 35 seconds at 38,000 feet. Thus, the period of useful consciousness was found to be approximately three-fourths of the total time during which consciousness was retained. Blood oxygen saturations averaged 64% at the appearance of the first error and 56% at the time of imminent unconsciousness.

Houston and Nez reported in December, 1945 on the relation of pulmonary ventilation to arterial oxygen saturation, (Pensacola, Project X675). In this study, it was found that arterial oxygen saturation is extremely sensitive to even small changes in pulmonary ventilation. Increasing of the resting volume by 30 to 50%, a change of which the subject is scarcely aware, will raise the arterial oxygen saturation 10 to 20%. Doubling or tripling the resting ventilation results in only a small further increase in saturation. Thus, for emergency breathing of air at moderate altitudes, doubling the resting ventilation will yield almost all the arterial oxygen saturation gain obtainable by any degree of ventilation and at the same time cause little acapnia. In a second report on this project, it was found that, in resting subjects breathing 10.5% O_2, the arterial oxygen tension bears a direct and linear relation to the respiratory minute volume although no arterial tensions were found to exceed the tracheal oxygen tension. A moderate amount of hyperventilation during this degree of anoxia increases arterial oxygenation and results in marked subjective improvement without recognizable symptoms of acapnia, at least during 15 minute periods. Under these experimental conditions, the increase in arterial oxygen tensions during hyperventilation is shown to be greater than the decrease in arterial carbon dioxide tension. Work on this problem is still continuing.

Smith and Pace in August, 1945, reported on the effect of acute hypoxia, with and without added CO_2, on the blood cells in man, (Project X313). They found that exposure of 29 individuals to lowered oxygen tension, (10% oxygen in nitrogen), for 20 minutes produced no immediate significant alterations in the mean values of white cell count, red cell count, hematocrit, hemoglobin concentration or red cell volume. Addition of carbon dioxide to give a range of 2 to 5% carbon dioxide in the low oxygen mixture did not alter these measurements. Work on this project is continuing.

In Project X524, Pace, Consolazio, and Lozner at the Naval Medical Research Institute worked on the transfusion of human erthrocytes as a possible means of increasing tolerance to hypoxia. A total of 1300 ml. of 55% fresh erythrocyte suspension in saline was administered intravenously to each of two subjects over a period of three days. The transfusions were well tolerated, causing only mild symptoms. The hematocrit reading was increased from 45.8% to 52.7% in one subject and from 50.0% to 56.1% in the other subject, representing an increase of approximately 12% in the total cell volume. The increased hematocrit readings gradually returned to normal over a period of approximately one month; at the end of 12 days, the increase was still greater than half the peak value attained. Analysis of arterial blood samples taken at altitudes indicated that the percentage saturation of hemoglobin with oxygen was within the normal range for the ambient oxygen partial pressure. Thus, the oxygen content of the blood, as well as the oxygen capacity, was greater than normal at this altitude. In tests made at simulated altitude of 18,000 feet to determine any deviation from normal reaction, the subjects, who were experienced in low pressure work subjectively noted an improved tolerance to hypoxia during the several days of maximum polycythemis. Work along these lines is still continuing.

In January, 1945, Weatherby and Burt reported from Pensacola on an evaluation of complete inspiratory obstruction as a warning of failure of oxygen supply to a demand regulator, (Project X500). They concluded that complete inspiratory obstruction appears to consitute a positive warning of oxygen supply failure whether the failure occurs suddenly or gradually. Any oxygen regulator changes designed to afford this warning should provide for the maintenance of the proper air-oxygen mixture up to the point of complete inspiratory obstruction lest anoxia, with its associated mental confusion and perhaps unconsciousness, obscure this warning. With the Pioneer diluter demand regulator, at altitudes above 25,000 feet, danger of insufficient oxygen supply resulting from low pressure, without warning, probably does not exist.

In Project X616, the Altitude Training Unit at the Naval Air Station, Norfolk, tested aviation personnel to obtain their reaction to inspiratory obstruction at simulated altitude. Exposing 50 naval aviators w thout warning to inspiratory obstruction resulting from an induced failure of the oxygen supply at 30,000 feet simulated altitude, they found that all of the subjects within 17 plus or minus 2 seconds were certain of the time when the obstruction took place. This was considered tantamount to an immediate warning of oxygen failure. All subjects showed anxiety at the sudden increased resistance to breathing. Trained subjects were able to handle the situation adequately while untrained subjects showed signs of varying degrees of mental confusion.

From this study, the Norfolk group suggested that an oxygen regulator equipped with an automatic device to warn aviators of loss of oxygen should be developed.

OXYGEN

Physiology - Pressure Breathing

Development of Pressure Breathing

The Navy's part in the development of pressure breathing equipment is somewhat incidental to that of the Army and civilian loboratories. However, certain phases of this problem were studied at the Naval Medical Research Institute and the Naval Air Experimental Station, Philadelphia. The work at Philadelphia, under Project X631, resulted in the adoption by the naval service of a unique combination of pressure breathing oxygen regulator and bail-out equipment developed by Gressly. A limited number of these devices are being used for high altitude flights by naval aircraft.

As a corollary of the development of the equipment described above, the Aero Medical Department, Naval Air Experimental Station, Philadelphia, has been a clearing agency for the indoctrination and training of pilots in the use of pressure breathing equipment. This work is still continuing.

One phase of pressure breathing may be termed almost exclusively a Navy development. This is the so-called emergency breathing procedure, (EBP), or "voluntary pressure breathing". This was developed first on an empirical basis by Commoner at the Naval Air Station, Corpus Christi, and was subsequently the object of a great amount of experimental work in other Navy and civilian laboratories. This procedure, as the name implies, was designed as an emergency maneuver for use in the event of failure of the oxygen supply at altitudes up to 25,000 feet and was demonstrated in flight as well as in the low pressure chamber. According to the original procedure, it was considered advantageous to exert pressure by contracting the respiratory muscles while holding a deep breath. As a result of subsequent investigations, doubt was cast on the value of exerting this pressure; these studies showed that at least a major portion of the beneficial effects resulted from hyperventilation. This question of the mechanism of the effect has not been resolved completely, however, and is incidental to the practical application of the procedure.

Owing to the effect which official promulgation of this maneuver might have on oxygen discipline, the only general dissemination made of this knowledge consisted of information appearing in the Aviation Supplement of the Bureau of Medicine and Surgery News Letter. While this may indicate to some that this development was of minor importance, it should be emphasized that Commoner's original work stimulated a considerable amount of valuable physiological work on the mechanism of the effects of anoxia on man.

Specific Projects

In October, 1943, Commoner at Corpus Christi, in Project X198, developed a "Training Manual for the Emergency Breathing Procedure". In work leading up to the preparation of this manual, he found that voluntary pressure breathing of air increases the aviator's physiological ceiling by approximately 10,000 feet and thus could enable an aviator, without equipment of any kind, to maintain an alert, conscious condition at altitudes of 25,000 to 26,000 feet for periods of as long as 30 minutes. He found that this procedure could successfully be taught to aviators by means of a supervised training run in a low pressure chamber. When the procedure was properly carried out, Commoner felt that there were no dangers from hyperventilation or other physiological hazards. This pressure breathing procedure could be useful in sustaining aviators at high altitudes in emergenciss, during parachute falls from high altitudes, and as an emergency procedure in aircraft pressurized cabins. Using pressure breathing of 100% oxygen, he found that an altitude of 40,000 feet could be reached with ordinary oxygen equipment and that possibly the physiological ceiling could be raised to approximately 50,000 feet. This manual written by Commoner was never used as an official training manual but was distributed to other research activities for information only.

In June, 1944, Commoner's group made actual flight tests at an indicated altitude of 25,000 feet for 10, 18, 21, 24, and 26 minutes. Co-pilots were able to maintain the aircraft on instruments, and the radioman functioned successfully, all without oxygen. One individual was able to recover from anoxia after its onset. From this test, Commoner reiterated his belief that his procedure could be very valuable in emergencies at 25,000 feet without oxygen. In July, 1944, Commoner reported that hyperventilation is not an adequate means of survival without oxygen at 25,000 feet since most subjects collapse from anoxia, acapnia, or both within eight minutes. Hyperventilation achieves an arterial oxygen saturation of only 65 to 79% at this altitude and is even more dangerous than normal breathing of air. Thus, in Commoner's opinion, the emergency breathing procedure remains the only effective and practical means of surviving, without oxygen, high altitude emergencies of tactical significance.

In this same project, No. X198, and in Project X454, Gemmill, Lilienthal, and Riley at Pensacola took a stand differing somewhat from that of Commoner. They concluded that pressure breathing in a normal atmosphere increased "altitude tolerance" by approximately 4,000 feet as estimated by the oxygen saturation of the arterial blood at 42,000 feet and 43,000 feet but that evidence could not be considered sufficient for a quantitative estimate of the increase in "altitude tolerance". The increase in oxygen saturation of the arterial blood during pressure breathing at altitude reflects the maximum rise in partial pressure of alveolar oxygen produced by the pressure breathing although this pressure obtains only during 2/5 of the respiratory cycle. In a second report, they felt that the effect of pressure breathing upon the arterial oxygen saturation is explained adequately by the increase in mean intrapulmonary pressure, (which is increased by pressure breathing by more than 100 mm.Hg.).

This Pensacola group agreed with Commoner that pressure breathing does increase altitude tolerance and, therefore, might prove useful in certain specific emergencies, but they pointed out several real dangers and difficulties inherent in the use of pressure breathing by air crews: (a) the development in some instances of severe degrees of acapnia (even tetany) due to hyperventilation; (b) the inadequate respiratory coordination in some individuals, with resultant impairment of "altitude tolerance"; (c) the difficulties involved in indoctrinating large groups of men and furthermore, the question of insuring that men maintain efficiency in performing the technique; (d) the possible development of over-confidence in an emergency maneuver which might encourage attempts to fly at hazardous altitudes without oxygen. These latter objections were the main reasons for not promulgating widespread service use of the voluntary pressure breathing method.

In Project X291, King, Goldman, Henson and Whaley at the Naval Medical Research Institute, in June, 1944, made a physiological appraisal of voluntary pressure breathing. They concluded, from tests at 25,000 feet, that no advantage is gained by application of pressure during hyperventilation, and that the emergency breathing procedure and voluntary hyperventilation are equally effective in increasing the oxygen saturation of arterial blood when breathing ambient air at simulated altitudes of 18,000 to 20,000 feet. On the basis of their work, they doubted whether a large percentage of flight personnel would be able to attain the required degrees of proficiency in voluntary pressure breathing without intensive training.

In Project X343, voluntary pressure breathing was again evaluated by Houston, Nuzie, Seitz, and Besson at the Naval Air Station, Miami. They concluded that while the precedure would have merit in prolonging consciousness of a subject, breathing air at 25,000 feet, it was difficult to learn and to perform except under the most favorable circumstances. They found that subjects had difficulty in performing EBP while attempting even simple tasks and tended to sacrifice EBP to complete their tasks, with severe anoxia ensuing. For these reasons, they considered EBP impractical for aviation personnel. In a later report, they concluded that hyperventilation at the rate of 12 to 15 breaths per minute is easier and less fatiguing than EBP at the same rate, and equally effective.

J. PHARMACOLOGY

In Project X213, at Camp Lejeune, Corey and Webster checked the effects of scopolamine on marksmanship and found that men given this drug performed with equal efficiency, both before and after its administration.

In February, 1943, Corey and Webster checked the effects of benzedrine on "fire power" (hits per minute) under conditions of extreme fatigue (Project X120). They found that 10 mgm. doses at 8-hour intervals, significantly increased fire power of personnel subjected to ardous tasks; they observed slight degrees of euphoria and diminished judgment.

Further reference to pharmacology problems appears in the sections on Motion Sickness, Vision, and Oxygen.

K. PHYSICAL FITNESS

While "physical fitness" was not the object of any intensive investigation by Naval Aviation Medical personnel, a large-scale program of physical training was conducted in pre-flight and flight schools. Critical analyses of the Schneider index and similar "condition"-evaluating indices were made with no sufficiently definite conclusions being found to justify changing the present aviation physical examination.

In Project X709 at Pensacola, Patterson is developing a Physical Fitness Test to establish standards of fitness for Naval Personnel.

L. SAFETY DEVICES AND SURVIVAL-HUMAN FACTORS IN ENGINEERING DESIGN

General Summary

In a sense, all of the research in aviation medicine described in other sections has as its fundamental purpose an increase in the safety and efficiency of flying personnel. However, certain specific aspects of the problem were attacked directly in the form of (a) surveys of the human factors concerned in aircraft accidents and (b) fundamental studies aimed toward determination of the forces which can be withstood by various structures in the body during abrupt deceleration.

With regard to the human factors involved in flying and the possible causes for aircraft crashes, medical personnel assigned to the Office of Flight Safety, Bureau of Aeronautics, and the Medical Liaison officers in Military Requirements Division, Bureau of Aeronautics, took an active part in an accident prevention program. A group at the Marine Corps Air Station, Cherry Point, prepared an admirable summary of the human factors involved in aircraft crashes, insofar as these could be assayed, and the nature of injuries sustained in relation to the condition of the airplane and the crash.

The School of Aviation Medicine at the Naval Air Training Bases, Pensacola, carried out a series of fundamental studies on the possible causes of disorientation in pilots, especially under conditions of night flying. This study has led to rather unexpected findings concerning the relationship of ocular movements to slow angular accelerations and has, in a sense, opened a new field of fundamental research. This work was carried forward by Graybiel in particular and is reported in the section on Orientation in Flight.

A fundamental study of the anatomical and physiological factors to be considered in engineering design was initiated early in 1945 by the Aviation Branch, Research Division and the Naval Medical Research Institute, in cooperation with the Special Devices Division, Office of Research and Inventions. This project is still continuing and is aimed toward standardization of aircraft cockpits in terms of functional design rather than of engineering convenience. Anthropological measurements and human factors, such as the optimal placing or critical controls, are already being incorporated in mock-ups of proposed new airplanes. An annotated bibliography, "Human Factors in Engineering Design", was prepared by Lawrence and Macmillan, Aviation Branch, Research Division, Bureau of Medicine and Surgery. It will be made available to all concerned with the design and development of new aircraft. It is not possible to estimate the number of aircraft crashes which might have been prevented had human factors been taken into consideration in the design of cockpits available in military aircraft during the war. However, it cannot fail to be considerable.

The first phases of fundamental studies of the decelerative and accelerative forces which can be withstood by various structures of the body have been carried out at the Naval Medical Research Institute, using the impact decelerator. The information so obtained will be checked by means of a split tube catapult, crashing of stricken aircraft and the like, using anthropological dummies, animals, and, finally, human volunteers.

Fundamental data have been gathered on factors involved in escape from aircraft. While the Navy has done relatively little experimental work in this field, much time has been spent on surveys and calculations to assay the possibility of escape under a variety of conditions. Partly as a result of these studies, the Bureau of Aeronautics and the Office of Research and Inventions are undertaking the construction of equipment for the development of ejection seats and a large human centrifuge at the Aero Medical Department, Naval Air Experimental Station, Philadelphia. Much of this work which was initiated during the war will not bear fruit unless adequate support is obtained for aviation medical research.

Air-Sea Rescue

Specific details regarding the various projects bearing on the provision of emergency food and water, and related items, have been discussed separately. However, the general aspects of the development of the air-sea rescue program warrant discussion as an entity.

The circumstances leading to the need for such a program are too well known to be enumerated. As part of the organization of "Dumbo" units, the operation of crash boats, etc., naval aviation medical personnel played an active part in the development of airborne equipment to aid in the handling of survivors. Specifically, improved litters, hoists, droppable rafts, first aid kits, and methods of packaging medical supplies for dropping to survivors, were perfected by cooperative efforts of engineering and medical personnel. In 1944, the Air-Sea Rescue Agency formally established a committee to study the medical and physiological aspects of air-sea rescue. Representatives of the Army, Navy, Coast Guard and Public Health Service met at frequent intervals to coordinate their efforts to establish an effective organization. In addition to these meetings, naval personnel participated in several survey trips of air-sea rescue facilities throughout the various operational areas.

Specific studies at naval aviation activities, and other branches of the Service, include sunburn protective ointments, life preservers, especially with regard to the optimal flotation position in the event of unconsciousness, prevention or alleviation of immersion foot, shark repellents, optimal positions to be taken by personnel during ditching, protection against underwater blast, testing of various signalling devices, and the use of oxygen equipment for emergency escape from submerged or submerging aircraft. These are in addition to research described in the sections of this report dealing with Food and Water, and Clothing.

Representatives of naval aviation medical activities aided in the training of "aviation equipment and survival officers", the organization of this training program originating from the Naval Air Training Bases, Pensacola.

The part played by aviation medical personnel, in the preparation of numerous survival manuals, has been described in the section on Food and Water.

Specific Projects

In 1943, aircraft Crash Investigation Boards were set up in various operational commands, with medical and engineering personnel as members, to investigate crashes and the causes thereof, and to correlate structural damage to aircraft with physical injuries to personnel. Standard report forms for recording the results of investigations were adopted and made available for statistical analysis of crashes. This work was done in conjunction with Project X115.

In March, 1944, Gemmill and co-workers at Pensacola made a comparison of different types of parachute harnesses, with particular reference to ease of release (Project X292). They compared standard Navy and British "quick release" harnesses. In the majority of cases, the British type harness was released with greater speed and ease than was the standard Navy type. However, the danger of accidental jamming, and possibly of accidental release, was considered much greater with the British than with the Navy type harness.

In May, 1944, Shelesnyak and Margolis at the Naval Medical Research Institute designed an individual personal first aid kit for aviation personnel (Project X371). This was planned to afford a compact plastic container with properties of moisture resistance, shock and abrasion protection, and to contain a sufficient quantity of essential first aid materials for one individual until more complete help could be obtained. Shelesnyak in April, 1945, devised a compact first aid kit for aeronautic pneumatic life rafts, (Project X554).

Turner, at the Naval Medical Research Institute, tested cardboard splints which had been submitted for evaluation (Project X447). He found them unsatisfactory because they burned readily and failed under conditions simulating tropical rain.

Grossman at Pensacola, in May of 1945, prepared three types of medical kits for air-sea rescue missions (Project X557). These were constructed so as to be readily portable and so that any item of equipment could be removed without disturbing any other items.

Jennings and co-workers at the Naval Medical Research Institute have devised various new stretchers, and modifications of old stretchers, under Project X109. These improvements consist of harnesses for carrying the patient in a vertical position in cases where such transportation is necessary; of flotation devices to support the patient on his stretcher in the water; and of emergency flotation and carrying devices to be used in place of standard equipment where the same is not available. Although none of these devices has yet been adopted as standard equipment, trials and evaluations of them are still being carried out in the field.

Under Projects X691 and X707, the Naval Medical Research Institute and the Submarine Base, New London, are working on improvements in life preservers to determine flotation characteristics, such as angle of the body from the horizontal, height of head above water line, and speed of turning from face-down to face-up position. This study, when completed, should give valuable information regarding the best equipment to support subjects (including unconscious ones) in the water.

Under Project X630, the Naval Medical Research Institute has been investigating crash injuries and protective measures against, studying the biomechanics of injury on a quantitative basis for the development of devices and procedures for protection of personnel. In August, 1945, Bierman reported on static loading tests of lap safety belts and shoulder harnesses (NAF-1201-1). He found that breakage in the shoulder harness assembly invariably occurred in the metal parts at a load of approximately 850 pounds, while the failure of the lap safety belts occurred at the metal parts under loads of approximately 2500 pounds. He concluded that the metal fittings of these belts and harnesses are the weakest components and recommended that the metal fittings should be made to withstand at least the loads accepted by the webbing (1355 lb. for the shoulder harness and 3150 lb. for the lap belt). In further work on other belts and harnesses, Bierman applied static loads to the point of failure, finding that while these assemblies met Navy specifications, their strength would not be adequate if the seats to which they were attached were constructed to withstand higher loads.

An impact decelerator was designed by Bierman to apply an impact force to a human being through aircraft shoulder straps and seat belts, simulating somewhat aircraft crash conditions. This device is limited by the abnormal position of the subject, by the fact that the restraining mechanism rather than the individual is accelerated, and by the restriction of visceral movement afforded by the apparatus.

Bierman and Larsen used this apparatus to investigate the distribution of impact pressures transmitted to the human body through the regulation shoulder straps and seat belt of aircraft. They found that the seat belt exerts a maximal impact pressure to the body at the umbilicus through the center of the belt, and that the shoulder straps exert their maximal impact pressures at the clavicular areas. They concluded that "an improved design of the present restraining devices in aircraft, allowing a more equal distribution of the impact pressures on the body, may permit increased tolerance to such pressures".

In additional future investigations under this project, it is planned to study deceleration forces in crashed airplanes, using anthropological dummies, animals, and, if practicable, human volunteers.

Under Project X716, Webster, Biodynamics Branch, Research Division, Bureau of Medicine and Surgery, is working on the physiological limits of escape from aircraft, with particular emphasis on high velocity and high altitudes. Methods of escape will be evaluated, together with existing data on physiological limits and human tolerance to acceleration and deceleration, anoxia, cold, etc. Calculation will be made of the physical stress imposed on the body by airplanes flying at high speeds and high altitudes, and of the stresses imposed by various methods of escape from aircraft. These physical and physiological findings will be correlated in order to set the limits for velocity and altitude at which flying can be recommended, and to recommend possible methods of escape from aircraft at high altitudes and high velocities.

In Project X647, Webster, Biodynamics Branch, Research Division, Bureau of Medicine and Surgery, is working on altitude, velocity and time relationships for free falls and parachute descents from aircraft. Tables have been prepared for determining times and rates of descent from any altitude to any other altitude for free falls and parachute jumps. These data will be correlated with the times of total and useful consciousness an aviator will have on "bailing out" at any given altitude with and without oxygen. Limits of safety as regards anoxia, cold, deceleration and duration of descents will be formulated.

In Project X677, the Marine Corps Air Station at Cherry Point is making an extensive investigation of safety factors in escape from aircraft. No report on this work has been submitted as yet.

In Project X695 the Pensacola group are making an analysis of a random sample of Navy air-sea rescues. This work, when reported on, should be valuable in evaluating present methods of air-sea rescue and in suggesting future improvements.

M. SPEECH INTELLIGIBILITY

Specific Projects

In September, 1943, Steer, working at Pensacola, evaluated the inter-communication systems used in Navy planes at that time, and recommended changes for improvement (Project X123). This same worker in Project X322 devised a new gosport speaking tube for training planes and found it to be definitely superior to the standard issue gosport. He recommended adoption of the new device.

Steer, Hadley and Kerr, in Project X520, prepared a series of recordings designed for training of primary flight students in the techniques of accurate listening and of improved inter-communication. These recordings were found to be of definite aid to primary flight students in that portion of their training involving the following of directions of flight instructors.

This same group of workers under Project X634 found the Gleason gosport mouthpiece to be definitely superior to Navy standard issue. They recommended its adoption by the service.

Under Project X645 Steer, Hadley and Kelly conducted extensive investigations on techniques to measure and evaluate speech intelligibility for flight personnel. They devised standard lists of terms to be used in flight instruction and, in addition, trained flight instructors in techniques of good voice transmission to insure audibility and intelligibility.

N. TOXIC GASES

General Summary

The principal toxic gas problems centered around the entrance of exhaust gases into the cockpit enclosures of naval aircraft. Certain necessary structural characteristics of carrier-based aircraft made this problem somewhat more serious in naval planes than in Army-type planes. Also, the Navy placed more emphasis upon toxic gas problems, in part because of the length of patrol flights and the need for maximum visual performance.

In the early part of the war, very little was known about the effects of carbon monoxide on the body when exposure occurred at altitudes involving moderate degrees of anoxia. There was a tendency toward ultra-conservatism and limits that were almost beyond the range of any known detecting instruments were set by some branches of the service. For these reasons, two main lines of development were emphasi ed: (1) study of the physiological effects of carbon monoxide when combined with altitude anoxia, and (2) the development of instrumentation for measuring concentrations of this gas in air and blood.

In connection with phase (1) above, the major studies were accomplished at the School of Aviation Medicine, Pensacola, and at the Naval Medical Research Institute. The group at Pensacola used as their main tool changes in the critical frequency of flicker and showed that 8 to 10 percent carbon monoxide hemoglobin depresses altitude tolerance by 4,000 to 6,000 feet at altitudes around 10,000 feet. A great amount of work relative to the physiological effects of carbon monoxide at altitude was accomplished at the Naval Medical Research Institute resulting in a distinct contribution to this field of physiology. Their work concerned principally the altitude decrement attributable to given concentrations of carbon monoxide at various altitudes using measurements such as the pulse rate response to exercise, visual fields, body sway, critical flicker frequency, and more general measures of performance as criteria. They, together with Pensacola, and the Harvard Fatigue Laboratory groups showed that a very regular linear equation could be used for calculating the rate of uptake of carbon monoxide by the body. These data were presented in the form of a nomograph by which the expected blood concentration could be determined provided the air concentrations of CO altitude, and time of exposure were known.

As a result of the physiological work, outlined above, and with the cooperation of civilian laboratories, a more reasonable assay of the combined effects of altitude anoxia, and carbon monoxide anoxia, could be made. In addition, the Bureau of Medicine and Surgery recommended a complete change in policy regarding the methods for estimating carbon monoxide hazard in naval aircraft, so that the blood level, rather than the air concentration of CO, would be used as a standard. This policy has been adopted in principle by the Bureau of Aeronautics and provides a more logical basis for the acceptance or rejection of military aircraft.

As a corollary to the cockpit toxic gas problem, that of suitable ventilation of the hangar decks of aircraft carriers during the warm-up period was studied. To accomplish this, several teams from the Naval Medical Research Institute determined carbon monoxide concentrations in the air and in the blood of exposed personnel aboard carriers of various classes. As a result of these tests, procedures were established which provided ventilation by use of the propeller wash from the planes themselves. In addition, recommendations for modifications of the ships' ventilating system were made and these were applied in the construction of the USS MIDWAY.

In all of the above studies, it was necessary to determine whether or not there were any other substances in the exhaust from airplane engines which would add to the toxicity of the carbon monoxide. It was concluded that, while certain aldehydes might be a source of irritation, the toxicity of exhaust gases could be suitably evaluated on the basis of their carbon monoxide content alone.

The Navy played an important role in the development of improved methods for the determination of carbon monoxide. Most of the work pertaining to this determination in air was sponsored by the Bureau of Aeronautics and led to the adoption of the NBS Colorimetric Kit perfected by Dr. Martin Shephard, National Bureau of Standards, based on a British development, and led to the adoption of the heated Hopcalite carbon monoxide indicator, manufactured by the Mine Safety Appliances Company. These and other methods were tested by medical personnel at the Naval Medical Research Institute, Philadelphia, Pensacola, and especially at the Naval Air Training Center, Patuxent. A careful comparative evaluation of various methods for determining carbon monoxide in air was accomplished at the Naval Medical Research Institute. The evaluation of methods for determination of carbon monoxide in blood was done at Patuxent, the Naval Medical Research Institute and Pensacola. Special efforts were expended on perfection of the Scholander method and on simple photoelectric colorimeter types of apparatus, developed by the National Institute of Health and the Aero Medical Laboratory, Wright Field. For a considerable period, the Naval Medical Research Institute performed services in the analysis of blood samples from numerous activities.

Possible toxic gas problems pertaining to the use of rockets in aircraft were studied. This applied particularly to gases from jet assisted take-off units (JATO), since personnel on the flight deck were exposed to clouds of smoke from these units. Representatives from the Naval Medical Research Institute and the Research Division, Bureau of Medicine and Surgery, demonstrated the probable effects of these gases by static tests at the manufacturer's proving ground. No operational tests were conducted on carriers.

Another toxic gas which has received consideration, from an aviation standpoint, is methyl bromide. This gas, suggested for use in engine fire-extinguisher systems, has been avoided in naval aircraft until recently. Since it has considerable advantage over carbon dioxide as a fire extinguisher, at the recommendation of the Bureau of Medicine and Surgery, methods for warning of its presence in the atmosphere are being developed by the Bureau of Aeronautics. Existing recommendations provide that methyl bromide be used only in aircraft in which the engines are located at a considerable distance from inhabited spaces.

Specific Projects

In Project No. X129, Gemmill reported on the effects of blood concentrations of carbon monoxide on altitude tolerance. He concluded that subclinical anoxia, due to moderate altitude, added to subclinical anoxia of moderate COHb concentrations, may produce appreciable symptoms, which can be largely prevented by proper use of oxygen equipment. Even small increments in the concentration of COHb (8 to 10 percent) depresses "altitude tolerance" by 4,000 feet., or more, as measured by the flicker fusion test. Even at low pressure altitude and with low percentages of carbon monoxide in the atmosphere, prolonged periods of exposure may produce measurable reduction in "altitude tolerance".

In August, 1945, Lilienthal and Riley, in Project X409, reported on their study of the in vivo equilibrium between oxy-carboxy-, and reduced hemoglobin in blood of human subjects breathing gas mixtures containing from 0.005% to 0.015% carbon monoxide. They discovered that the amount of COHb could be determined from the Haldane equation, knowing only the percentage of CO in the inspired air and the pressure altitude. They found that the symptoms produced by CO are proportional not only to the blood concentration of COHb but also to the duration of exposure to given concentrations of CO.

Various groups of workers from the Naval Medical Research Institute studies ventilation problems in operating naval vessels, chiefly aircraft carriers and LST's carrying tanks (Project X154). The carbon monixide concentrations aboard these ships during plane and tank warm-ups were determined, and appropriate recommendations for controlling hazardous concentrations were made.

Workers at the Naval Air Station, San Diego, in March, 1944 (Project X361), reported on the carbon monoxide determinations in the F4U airplane. They found that, in the first 10 test flights, in unmodified F4U aircraft, all tests showed carbon monoxide, while 38 out of 48 readings were above the Navy limit. The highest concentrations were found when the aircraft was using either automatic rich or emergency rich carburetor mixture. They found that, on sealing the bulkhead aft of the pilot's compartment, these readings dropped to within safe limits.

The same group at the Naval Air Station, San Diego, compared the MSA portable Hopcalite carbon monoxide indicator and the bulb type colorimeter (Project X362). They concluded that the colorimeter has a possible error, as great as 0.007 percent, especially when dealing with small concentrations of carbon monoxide or readings below 0.005 percent. It is, however, excellent for use in cramped spaces in aircraft. They suggested research on its variability so that it could be more completely standardized.

Workers at the Naval Air Training Center, Patuxent and at the Naval Medical Research Institute conducted extensive investigations of determination of allowable safe limits of carbon monoxide concentrations in aircraft (Project X417). They introduced a continuous sampling device for gases in ambient air and evaluated existing methods for determining the concentration of carbon monoxide in air. They concluded that the iodine pentoxide train method is the most reliable but is limited to research laboratories as a standard of reference. The Bureau of Mines' apparatus is ideal for routine laboratory use but requires considerable specialized equipment, while the Beckman-McCullough method is the ideal one for use by naval activities since it is readily portable and requires only 15 minutes for an analysis. However, this latter device requires frequent calibration. The National Bureau of Standard's method was considered insufficiently accurate for aircraft acceptance tests. These workers constructed nomographs for the estimation of the uptake of carbon monoxide by the blood of flying personnel, for use while breathing air or breathing through a diluter demand regulator. These nomographs make estimation of the blood concentration of carbon monoxide readily available when the cockput concentration, altitude and exposure time are known.

Turner, Consolazio, and Gersh investigated the toxic gases resulting from jet-assisted takeoffs (JATO). They found that hydrochloric acid and carbon monoxide constitute the worst hazards to personnel exposed to jet-assisted takeoffs on carrier flight decks. These gases could create serious operational hazard if permitted to enter a ship's ventilating system. They suggested investigation of the hazards in actual tests aboard carriers.

In April, 1945, Lilienthal, at Pensacola, evaluated methods for analyzing blood concentrations of carbon monoxide (Project X555).

He found the AML instrument unsatisfactory in its original form but potentially very useful after an increase in accuracy. The National Institute of Health Midget Photometer was considered to be a very precise means for determining blood COHb.

The Naval Air Experimental Station, Philadelphia, reported in August, 1945, on a given MSA carbon monoxide indicator (Project X649). They concluded that without strict control measures, this instrument was liable to errors of 20 to 25 percent in determining carbon monoxide levels in air. It required frequent calibration and a standard carbon monoxide sample, and was vulnerable to breakdown or misuse in many stages between manufacturer and aircraft installation.

Further conclusions were that this indicator is unsatisfactory in its present form for Navy adoption. This same indicator was evaluated at Patuxent in Project X657 and similar conclusions were reached.

O. VISION

1. Aircraft and Instrument Lighting

Specific Projects

In September, 1942, Webster and Lee, working at the National Institute of Health, demonstrated the superiority of red lighting over fluorescent lighting for reading aeronautical charts and for preserving dark adaptation, (Project X69).

In May, 1945, Poppen reported from Corpus Christi, on his investigation of visual factors contributing to night aircraft accidents, (Project X498). As a result of a questionnaire submitted to 400 pilots, he determined that the greatest difficulties in night flying were confusion of lights, inability to judge speed and distance, and disorientation or vertigo. In a later report, he analyzed the times at night when accidents occurred at Corpus Christi. This study covered a period of 10 months in 1944. He found that the accident rate increased markedly as the evening advanced. This was shown to be not primarily due to increasing darkness because hours of essentially the same degree of darkness have decidedly different accident rates, nor could local changes in direction or velocity of the wind account for the increase in accident rate with the later hours. He felt that a reasonable hypothesis was that sleepiness and fatigue significantly increased in the later night hours and were probably responsible for the increased accident rate. Among suggested remedies, he advocated strict control of aviators to insure reasonable rest on the day in which night flying is to take place, and experimentation in aircraft lighting to determine the best system for avoiding disorientation.

Pfaffman, Fosberg and Bugelski in Project X562 corroborated Poppen's findings as to the increase in accident rate during the later night hours. This group also believed that the increase resulted from factors other than the level of illumination. They analyzed the accident rate in terms of the degree of illumination and concluded: (a) the total number of accidents is lower during periods of moonlight; (b) landing accidents involving low approaches occur less frequently in moonlight; and (c) accidents attributed to disorientation occur less frequently in moonlight. However, taxiing accidents occurred equally under moon and moonless conditions, and landing accidents attributed to leveling off too high tended to occur more frequently in moonlight.

Bromer, at the Naval Experimental Station, Philadelphia compared ultra-violet and indirect red systems of illumination for aircraft instrument panels (Project X636). He found that, when the brightness level was greater than that required for minimum legibility, ultra-violet illumination caused a sharp decrease in the efficiency of spotting faint targets against the sky background while the red system had very little effect. He therefore, recommended that red illumination be specified for Navy aircraft panel lighting.

2. Color Vision

Specific Projects

Early in the war, the source of supply for the Ishihara color plates was cut off from the Navy, and a new color test became imperative. Webster, in Project X34, evaluated the Inter-Society Color Council Color Vision Test at the Naval Aviation Cadet Selection Board, New York. This test, used 20 pairs of carefully devised colored chips, from each pair of which the subject chose the redder one. The test was found to be no better for diagnostic or screening purposes than the American Optical Company Pseudo-Isochromatic Plates (First Edition, 1940). Because of the much greater expense of the color chip test, it was decided that the AO plates would be the official color vision test for naval personnel. In further work evaluating these plates, it was decided to abridge the original 46 plates into a group consisting of those 20 plates with the greatest diagnostic significance, a passing score being 15 plates correctly read, regardless of color group. A recommendation embodying this change was made.

In February, 1943, Farnsworth on Project X42 reported from New London that the Canadian Navy Color Vision Lantern is an effective device for screening personnel. However, little was found to be gained by substituting this device for the pseudo-isochromatic plates. As a result of his study, Farnsworth decided to design a new lantern along lines similar to those of the Canadian device.

In Project X225, Farnsworth tested the Williams Lantern and found it to be entirely unsuited for Navy use.

Peckham, in Project X75, designed a new color perception test which was never officially adopted inasmuch as it offered no material advantage over previous methods.

In Project X348, Farnsworth studied the retention of hues at a distance. He found that a dark blue-green background (such as that offered by sea water) has little effect on the recognition of colors and that the color of the illumination (illuminant C and A) affects recognition of colors slightly.

Under Project X480, Naval Air Stations at Corpus Christi, Pensacola, Jacksonville and San Diego, the Submarine Base at New London, and Camp Lejeune compared the second edition of the American Optical Company Pseudo-isochromatic Plates with the first edition in general use. As a result of their reports, Aviation Branch, Research Division,

Bureau of Medicine and Surgery, recommended adoption of the second edition as the Navy standard, with changes to reduce the number of plates to 23, to make the passing score 16 correctly read plates, to eliminate the least diagnostic plate from each of the original group, and to administer the test under daylight or its equivalent in artificial illumination.

In Project X262, Farnsworth at New London discussed the relationship of illumination to the construction of pseudoOisochromatic plates. He stressed the necessity of using a standard illumination (such as the MacBeth Daylight Lamp), if the test is to be meaningful. He continued this work in Project X261.

In Project X502, Farnsworth checked the effect of tinted lenses on color vision. He found that neutral and greenish lenses produced little effect on color perception while reddish-orange lenses caused considerable effect, equivalent to that of moderate color blindness; yellow lenses produced the effect of extreme color blindness; and after-effects of wearing any colored lenses diminished rapidly.

Various projects are still underway to develop effective screening devices for color vision, to validate the Navy lantern developed at New London, to determine the critical hue regions of confusion for color-anomalous individuals, and to field-test men with varying degrees of color anomaly in specific Navy duties.

VISION

3. Vision Examination in the Aviation Physical Examination

Certain changes have been suggested in the vision testing portion of the aviation Form I examination. These suggestions have been submitted to various air stations for evaluation and may later be incorporated into changes in the examination as now carried out.

VISION

4. Vision, Miscellaneous

Specific Projects

Blum and Fishes at the Naval Medical Research Institute investigated the changes in visual fields under stress of naval conditions (Project X149). They concluded that the reduction in size of perimetric field observed in subjects exposed to prolonged physiologic stress, other than anoxia, is probably no greater than that observed under non-stress conditions. Acute anoxia, however, produces reversible reduction of the perimetric fields, apparently due to physiologic changes in the visual mechanism.

In July, 1944, Corey and Webster made a study at Camp Lejeune (Project X290), of marksmanship efficiency under conditions of low illumination. They concluded from test firing under low illumination that practical advantage is to be gained through the wearing of dark adapter goggles, through the illumination of targets by red as contrasted with white light, and through dilatation of the pupil by means of a mydriatic. They also found no correlation between rod threshold, as determined by the Navy Radium Plaque Adaptometer, and ability to score hits in reduced light.

McGehee at the Naval Air Station, Atlanta, evolved a technique for photographing the eye movements of pilots during instrument flight, (Project X170).

Patterson, Burt and Jones from Pensacola reported, in Project X541, on the effect of gravitational force (tilt table) on alteration of scotopic vision, and means of prevention of this effect. They found that progressive fall in blood pressure is associated with progressive impairment in visual acuity, this correlation being better in the case of the systolic and pulse pressures than in the case of the diastolic pressure. Under the conditions of their experiments, visual acuity measurements could not be used as indirect measures of blood pressure.

VISION

5. Night Vision

a. Dark Adaptation

Specific Projects

Webster, on the USS ENTERPRISE, using the Hecht-Shlaer adaptometer, studied the dark adaptation threshold of officers and men, finding no significant difference between them. All subjects who were deficient in original testing, improved on Vitamin A administration (Projects X20 and X21).

Webster, and Lee, working at the National Institute of Health, developed specifications for dark adaptation goggles for maximum dark-adapting effect (Project X22).

In Project X23, Lee and Webster, at the National Institute of Health, showed that the state of adaptation of one eye is to a large extent independent of the state of adaptation of the other eye, and that the resulting state of essentially monocular vision, under these circumstances, does not impair activity in simple motor situations. This phenomenon of the independence of dark adaptation of the two eyes is of value in situations where aviators flying at night may be suddenly exposed to any element which might tend to destroy dark adaptation. Merely closing one eye will protect the dark adaptation of that eye.

Lee, Fisher and Birren at the Naval Medical Research Institute reported on the effect on dark adaptation of varying intensities of illumination in ready rooms (Project X162). They found that the optimal lighting level for cone function in ready rooms for personnel wearing dark adaptation goggles was between 20 and 30 foot candles. Under this lighting level, the optimal time for dark adaptation, wearing the red goggles is 45 minutes, followed by 2 minutes of complete darkness. After exposure to light levels above 30 foot candles, an excessive amount of time was required to fully dark-adapt while levels below 20 foot candles gave insufficient illumination for cone function. If all-red lighting is used instead of the goggles, the intensity should be between 2.5 and 3.8 foot candles. This group also reported a wave-like fluctuation in the curve of dark adaptation with a 3 to 7 minute period and irregular amplitude of from 0.05 to 0.25 log units test brightness. They suggested further investigation of this fluctuation. In Project X211, Lee reported further on his investigation of rhythmic fluctuations appearing in dark adaptation curves.

Tousey, working at the Naval Research Laboratory, investigated the effect on night vision of radar screens of various colors and brightness (Project X196). In general, he found that green trace screens can be made satisfactory as regards night vision by the use of an orange filter and P-7 screens by means of a red filter.

In December, 1943, Lee compared the rates of dark adaptation under red illumination and in total darkness (Project X218). He found no measurable accelerating action resulting from exposure to red light. The thresholds obtained after red light exposure were higher than, or equal to, the corresponding thresholds following exposure to complete darkness.

Blum and Fisher reported on the determination of levels of illumination at which binocular fusion can take place (Project X254). They concluded from their experiments that any night vision training device should be binocular rather than monocular inasmuch as, at low illuminations, the perceptual threshold is lower for binocular than for monocular viewing, in most individuals.

Clark and Johnson, working at Pensacola in Project X439, reported in February, 1945, on the course of dark adaptation after wearing orange dark adapter goggles. They found that standard red goggles are markedly superior to 5% orange goggles and to 5 and 10% neutral goggles under conditions demanding quick recovery of complete dark adaptation. Where somewhat less complete recovery is required, the 5% orange goggles are almost as efficient as the standard red ones.

Peckham and Older, working at the Naval Air Station, Anacostia, (Project X483) concluded that black lenses do not permit any visual duties to be performed during the course of dark adaptation while red, orange, and gray lenses do permit visual duties. Of these latter, the red lenses are most useful in hastening dark adaptation but the orange lenses are more useful in allowing perception of some color.

Lee and Finch at the Naval Medical Research Institute, as a result of tests on wired goggles, reported that the wire heater element does not interfere significantly with night vision (Project X407).

Hecht, Hendley, Ross and Richmond, working at Camp Lejeune, in April 1945 reported on the effect of exposure to intense sunlight on subsequent night vision (Project X442). They concluded that exposure to ordinary sunlight produces temporary and cumulative effects on night vision. A single exposure of 2 to 3 hours delays the onset of rod dark adaptation by 10 minutes or more, and slows the process so that the normal night vision threshold is not reached for several hours. With repeated daily exposure to sunlight, the dealy in reaching the normal threshold persists overnight; this threshold, after complete dark adaptation, rises higher each day for about 10 days and then remains at the highest level. This elevated threshold corresponds to an average deterioration of about 50% in visual acuity, range of visibility, contrast discrimination, and in the frequency of picking up a barely visible target. This chronic effect does not disappear even after 10 days of protection from sunlight and is approximately equivalent to the loss in night vision suffered by flying at 12,000 feet at night without oxygen. These workers concluded that adequate sunglasses transmitting at the most 10 to 15%, should be used by all persons exposed to bright sunlight during the day who expect to perform critical night duties soon afterward. (See also the section on Protection of Vision.)

In Project X548, Lee reported that infrequent exposure of short duration to ultra-violet radiation from the lamp used by a landing signal officer will not appreciably impair dark adaptation. In Project X503, Orlansky, at Quonset Point, determined the effect of the Navy airborne search light on dark adaptation. He found the average recovery time on 174 runs to be 21.5 seconds with an average increase in instantaneous threshold of 0.49 log units.

VISION

Night Vision

b. Night Vision Scotometry

Specific Projects

Korb in July, 1945, reported the development of a diaphragm shutter scotometer for screening individuals with poor night vision (Project X529).

This scotometer was evaluated by Sulzman, working at New London (Project X492). He reported, in March, 1946, on the test-retest reliability of the Korb Scotometer and of the Livingston method of rod scotometry. He concluded that while the Korb Scotometer, in its original form, is not as reliable as other tests (Livingston screen, radium plaque at 5 feet and radium plaque at 7 feet), it is simple to operate, can be administered with rapidity, and appears to measure the same function. With improvement in mechanical difficulties and experimentation on a larger group of subjects, the Korb Scotometer gives promise of being a highly useful instrument.

VISION

Night Vision

C. Night Vision Testing

General Survey

During the early years of the war, it became evident that some test screening of individuals with poor night vision would have to be devised. Existing instruments for this purpose were found to be too complicated for routine service use, or to require too extensive laboratory investigation. Accordingly, there was developed the Navy Radium Plaque Adaptometer. Webster drew up the original plans for this adaptometer and Peckham devised the original model. Later, the device was officially adopted for Navy use and a program set up for training operators in its use. By Navy order, all naval personnel were required to take the test. After the Navy Radium Plaque Adaptometer testing program was adopted, it became further evident that training in the proper use of the eyes at night would be very valuable for Navy personnel and especially for aviators and lookouts. Various lookout training devices had been adopted by the Submarine Base at New London and found to be very effective. Wing Commander Evelyn of the Royal Canadian Air Force was consulted as to the use of his training device, and a demonstration was arranged by him at the Naval Auxiliary Air Station, Charles Town, early in 1944. Following this, the Navy decided to adopt the Evelyn device as a 2-dimensional means of demonstrating the principles involved in off-center vision, scanning, dark adaptation, etc. In addition to this, 3-dimensional models were procured for demonstrating actual terrain features, including both land and water, from simulated altitudes. These night vision training units were established at various air stations and used to indoctrinate aviation personnel in the techniques of night vision. In conjunction with this work, there was used a manual on "The Use of the Eyes at Night" which had been prepared in 1942 by Liljencrantz and Carson while on the Night Vision Board.

Specific Projects

In a series of projects, Numbers X24 through X29, various adaptometers were checked by Webster, Peckham and others for reliability and validity.

In Project X68, the New London group found test-retest data to be about 0.8 on both the NDRC II and the Radium Plaque Adaptometers, but inasmuch as the Radium Plaque Adaptometer was superior in construction and operation, its adoption by the naval service was recommended.

Lee and Fisher in Project X167 found the NDRC III adaptometer unsatisfactory.

Peckham and Verplanck conducted an extensive field test of the Radium Plaque Adaptometer at New London in 1943 and 1944 (Project X268). They determined that the critical pass score should be 16 correct responses out of 20 presentations and that additional trials would not improve the classification of men tested.

Macmillan and Commoner at Corpus Christi, in April, 1944 reported their conclusions that the Navy Radium Plaque Adaptometer was not sufficiently consistent to warrant its use as a selective device (Project X298). They suggested improvements in its design and instructions for use.

Ross, reporting from Camp Lejeune in Project X472, concluded that the Radium Plaque Adaptometer test at a 7-foot distance was a more useful and reliable test for classification than the standard Navy test and that the Radium Plaque Adaptometer at a 9-foot distance could be used for the rapid selection of individuals with superior night vision. In a later report, he found a significant degree of agreement between Radium Plaque Adaptometer scores and visual performance in the field, finding the score at 7 feet alone approximately as efficient as the total Radium Plaque Adaptometer score in predicting outdoor performance. He also found a high relationship between the Radium Plaque Adaptometer scores and the ability of subjects to detect silhouettes on the Evelyn night vision trainer.

Draeger, Lee and Fisher at the Naval Medical Research Institute, designed a new portable multiple brightness dark adaptometer (Project X311), which they found to be superior to the Radium Plaque Adaptometer in reliability, and equal to the modified Rostenberg adaptometer. Testing time per subject was approximately equal for the three adaptometers. Work on the multiple brightness adaptometer is continuing. The modified Rostenberg adaptometer, the Admiralty adaptometer, the Wright adaptometer, and the Beals Adaptometer have been studied in various projects (see appendix) and found to be unsuitable in one or more respects for Navy use.

VISION

Night Vision

d. Night Vision Training

Special Projects

Orlansky, at Quonset Point, reported favorably on the effect of night vision training (Evelyn Trainer) on Navy Radium Plaque Adaptometer scores (Project X558). He found that, following instruction on the Evelyn trainer, subjects made better scores originally and on retest on the Radium Plaque Adaptometer, than did subjects without the training. He suggested further studies on a larger population to validate these findings.

Clark and co-workers at Pensacola reported, in Project X563, on a study of the learning resulting from the use of the Navy night vision training device. They concluded that the night vision training demonstrations were much more effective in instructing aviation cadets on the principles and pitfalls of night vision than were routine lectures without training demonstrations.

Ross and Mueller at Camp Lejeune reported, in Project X582, that night vision training with the Evelyn trainer decreases the number of failures of the initial Radium Plaque Adaptometer test but has no significant effect on the group failure rate of subsequent tests.

VISION

6. Optical Instruments

Extensive trials of optical instruments have been conducted under field conditions at New London. This work has involved the use of binoculars, telescopes, range and sighting devices, and haze penetrating filters. Reports on this work have not as yet been compiled but, when furnished, they will provide extremely valuable information for Navy use.

7. Protection of Vision

Sun Glasses

The need for protecting the eyes of service personnel from extreme conditions of glare in the tropics and in Arctic regions was recognized early during the war. Various types of protective sun glasses were developed by the Navy and other laboratories under the sponsorship of the Army-Navy-OSRD Vision Committee. After much consultation and investigation, the Navy decided to sponsor neutral sun glasses of low transmission (10 to 15%) for general use, and of somewhat higher transmission (up to 30%) for aviation use. Polarization of these sun glasses was recommended for personnel other than aviators.

The Navy sun glasses type N-1 which were finally decided upon were checked by Clark, Johnson and Dreher at Pensacola for their effectiveness in protecting night vision (Project X561). They concluded that individuals who had previously been exposed to sunlight for extended periods daily for several months had lower night visual thresholds after being protected by these sun glasses than those who did not wear protective glasses. They reasoned that personnel wearing effective sun glasses during prolonged exposure to sunlight will have appreciably greater night visual efficiency than personnel not wearing them; hence, they advocated providing Navy personnel with these sun glasses routinely.

In Project X567 these same workers reported on the effect of excessive sunlight on the retinal sensitivity of an unprotected, and a completely protected eye in the same individual. They found that exposure of individuals, wearing a black eye shield over one eye, to excessive sunlight for several hours a day for a period of two weeks, produced a rise in the night visual threshold of the exposed eye over that of the protected eye. This emphasized a previous conclusion that personnel should be protected from excessive exposure to sunlight if night vision is to be maintained normally.

Ross and Mueller, at Camp Lejeune, studied the durability of Navy sun glasses, Type N-1, Project X583. They found considerable damage to result from relatively short periods of use, chiefly because of scratching of the plastic lenses.

Sun Scanning Glasses

Two types of sun scanning glasses were devised during this war. One type consisted of variable density polarizing goggles; the second type being fusion density goggles constructed by placing semi-opaque filters over the portions of the lenses used in direct viewing of the sun. The variable density glasses enable subjects to look directly at the sum but prohibit viewing the area around the sun. Fusion density glasses make viewing of the area immediately around the sun practicable.

Aviation Goggles

Improvements have been made in aviation goggles, both in those with plastic lenses and in those with glass lenses. Research is being conducted in plastics which are more resistant to scratching and which have anti-fogging properties. These goggles have become increasingly popular with aviators because of their comfort, wide field of vision and their easily replaced lenses for day use, protection against glare, and for dark adaptation.

Glass lenses for aviation goggles are being improved by providing neutral glass filters developed largely through the efforts of Peckham in collaboration with glass manufacturers. Availability of such neutral glass will be largely increased to provide for future Navy needs.

Ultra-Violet Protection

To protect the eyes of landing signal officers from the effects of ultra-violet light used to illuminate their suits and signal paddles, there was developed a non-fluorescent polarizing goggle (Projects X648 and X658).

VISION

8. Radiant Energy

Specific Projects

Peckham, in Project X453, discussed the protection of vision of aviation personnel against ultra-violet radiation. This problem becomes more and more important as higher altitudes are attained, increasing by a factor probably as great as 4 times. He suggested using either a special yellowish dye developed by the Polaroid Corporation or a Monsanto plastic insert in the transparent panels enclosing cockpits.

Blum at the Naval Medical Research Institute has devised tables and curves for calculating the energy transmission of sun glasses required for adequate protection of the retina from temporary and permanent damage from solar radiation (Project X435).

VISION

9. Stereoscopic Vision (Depth Perception)

In May 1942, Naval Reserve Aviation Base, Philadelphia, in collaboration with the Johnson Foundation Staff, evaluated a vectographic test of stereoscopic vision, finding it unsatisfactory (Project X33). Channel and Fontaine attempted to validate the Stromberg-Gwathmey test of depth perception, (Project X130). They fould that, although it had fair reliability, it had insufficient validity as a predictor of success in flight training to warrant its use in the selection of aviation cadets.

Trumbull at Pensacola is at present conducting an investigation of the reliability of the Verhoeff test of depth perception (Project X717).

VISION

10. Vision Testing

Special Projects

In November, 1944, Wolpaw and Imus investigated the vectographic device developed by the American Optical Company (Project X468). They found it insufficiently developed or standardized for accurate visual acuity and heterophoria determinations.

In Project X499, Wolpaw and Imus compared the Ortho-Rater with clinical ophthalmic examinations. In general, they found the battery of visual tests in this device to be as reliable as the clinical tests. For details of their findings, the original report should be consulted.

In Project X493, the New London group compared various screening devices with standard medical procedures. They concluded that the American Optical Sight Screener and the Bausch and Lomb Ortho-Rater were approximately equal in validity and reliability, while the Keystone Telebinocular was inferior in both respects. Their extensive findings can best be appreciated by consulting the original report. A further report in this project comprises a comparative study of various measures of heterophoria. The Maddox Rod method for measuring heterophoria was found to best satisfy critical requirements. Screening devices were concluded to be apparently as reliable as the clinical method for measuring heterophoria but the results do not correlate well. Further research is indicated to establish why there is no greater correspondence between the clinical and instrument measures.

Extensive investigation of the problem of visual acuity measurement regarding types of test objects, factors of illumination, brightness and contrast, and job analysis involving the fitting of specific visual skills to specific jobs, is being carried out under the auspices of the Army-Navy-NRC Vision Committee. At present, the Army is engaged in large scale testing of visual acuity targets. The results of this investigation may necessitate changes in the routine testing of vision of service personnel.

IV. LIST OF APPARATUS AND PROCEDURES ADOPTED AS A RESULT OF AVIATION MEDICAL RESEARCH

Development and testing of anti-G protection devices.

Study of physiological effects of rapid ascent to high altitude for establishment of criteria for advanced type aircraft.

Development of new micro techniques for visualization of aeroembolism in living tissues.

Development of pre-oxygenation techniques for prevention of divers' bends and aeroembolism in aviators.

Establishment of human breathing patterns at sea level and altitude for use in design of aviators' oxygen breathing equipment.

Flight testing and evaluation of Navy aircraft oxygen regulators.

Establishment of criteria for design of Bureau of Aeronautics oxygen equipment.

Development of a simple flowmeter type apparatus for testing oxygen regulators in aircraft.

Establishment of standards for size distribution of A-14 oxygen mask for use by naval personnel.

Comparative tests of devices for testing of high altitude oxygen mask leakage leading to modification of existing equipment.

Development of procedure for instruction and indoctrination of key aviators in problems of high altitude flight and pressure oxygen breathing equipment.

Evaluation of techniques employed in oxygen indoctrination of aviation personnel.

Development and evaluation of voluntary pressure breathing methods and techniques.

Development of new simple methods for blood gas analysis.

Investigation and recommendations regarding dental pain occurring in flight.

Evaluation of visual standards for use in selection of naval aviators.

Development of aptitude tests for selection of naval aviators.

Development of aptitude tests for the selection of flight instructors.

Development of aptitude tests for the selection of aircraft gunners.

Development of improved techniques in aircraft inter-communication systems.

Development of improved techniques in speech intelligibility of communication in aircraft.

Development of an emergency ration for life rafts.

Development of protective anti-sun headgear for life rafts.

Evaluation of motion sickness preventives for use in life raft first-aid kits, leading to recommendations for adoption of scopolamine.

Development of individual first-aid kit for flying personnel.

Development of techniques for dropping of medical supplies from aircraft.

Development of improved naval in-flight rations.

Development of special methods for interior and exterior lighting of aircraft.

Establishment of method of illuminating submarine conning towers.

Determination of and recommendation of methods for elimination of factors causing disorientation in pilots during flight at night.

Establishment of criteria based on human factors in the design, placement, and operation of instruments and controls in aircraft, and pilot comfort, efficiency and escape.

Preparation, compilation and editing of a 220 page book entitled, "Annotated Bibliography on Human Factors in Engineering Design".

Development of nylon aviator's flak suit.

Evaluation of crash injuries, leading to establishment of methods for prevention.

Development of harness for protection against crash deceleration, and parachute opening shock.

Testing and recommendations for improvement of ventilation on naval aircraft and aircraft carriers.

Recommendations based on the investigation of toxic gases produced by JATO units.

Development of single aperture goggle for uninterrupted, wide-angle vision.

Development of red goggles for dark adaptation.

Development of radium plaque adaptometer for night vision testing.

Development of brow-rest all-purpose Navy sun glasses.

Development of sun-scanning visor for ground, ship, and flying personnel.

Research leading to the establishment of specifications for aviators' neutral sun glasses.

Development of equipment for indoctrination of naval personnel in techniques to aid in night vision.

Recommendation for methods of prevention of deleterious effects, on subsequent night vision, of exposure to intense sunlight.

Development of anti-fluorescent goggle to prevent dazzling of landing signal officer.

Development of new color vision test book.

Development of new Navy color vision testing lantern.

Development of a field method for the measurement of the central scotoma under dim illumination.

Development and evaluation of test targets for measuring visual acuity.

Evaluation of the Orthorater, Sight-screener, and Telebinocular as compared to standard methods of visual testing.

Evaluation of binoculars, leading to recommendation of those best suited for naval use.

Preparation, compilation and editing of a 109 page book entitled, "A Bibliography of Aviation Medicine Supplement".

V. APPENDIX

LIST OF PROJECTS AND REPORTS BY SUBJECTS

A. ACCELERATION

1. X-1 - Flight testing of anti-blackout equipment prior to fleet testing. (Anacostia)

   - Report in letter form to BUMED, ANTI-BLACKOUT EQUIPMENT - TEST OF, 27 April 1942. (Ferwerda)

   - Report - NAVY ANTI-BLACKOUT SUITS AND ATTACHMENTS, 14 October 1942. (Carson and Ferwerda) Report in letter form to BUAER, copy to BUMED, ANTI-BLACKOUT EQUIPMENT, GRADIENT PRESSURE TYPE, CENTRIFUGE TEST OF, 16 October 1942. (Ferwerda)

   - Report in letter form to BUAER, copy to BUMED, ANTI-BLACKOUT EQUIPMENT, SUMMARY AND PRESENT STATUS OF, 11 December 1942. (Ferwerda)

2. X-71 - Tolerance to acceleration. (Pensacola)

   - Report dated 26 March 1943, HIGH ACCELERATIONS IN INTERMEDIATE TRAINING: INCIDENCE OF SYMPTOMS AND AN ESTIMATE OF TOLERANCE TO "G". (School of Aviation Medicine)

3. X-98 - Fleet test of anti-blackout equipment. (Jacksonville)

   - Report in letter form to Anacostia from Cecil Field. Subject: ANTI-BLACKOUT EQUIPMENT: REPORT OF, 11 November 1942. (Konrad)

4. X-610 - Bibliography on acceleration. (Pensacola)

   - Report No. 1, ANNOTATED BIBLIOGRAPHY ON THE PHYSIOLOGICAL EFFECTS OF ACCELERATION IN AIRCRAFT, 1 September 1945. (Burt)

5. X-693 - Study of high accelerations. (Pensacola)

6. X-723 - Methods for calculation of forces acting on the human being in flight and in the centrifuge. (Pensacola) No report, work continuing.

7. TED NAM 25640 - BLADDERS - VINYLITE COATED NYLON - ANTI-BLACKOUT SUITE - INDURANCE TEST OF, 20 February 1945. (NAES, PHILADELPHIA)

8. TED NAM 25712 - Report on ANTI-BLACKOUT EQUIPMENT - INVESTIGATION DEVELOPMENT AND TEST OF, 3 April 1946. (NAES, Philadelphia, Watts)

9. TED PTR 25104 - Report on TEST OF QUICK DISCONNECT COUPLINGS OF ANTI-BLACKOUT EQUIPMENT, 18 October 1945, 25104.1. (NATC, Patuxent River)

B. CLOTHING

1. X-128 - Comparative testing of electrically heated flying suits, (Taylor suit versus U. S. Navy suit). (Pensacola)

- Report - Same title as above, 20 July 1943. (School of Aviation Medicine)

2. X-189 - Protective clothing for subjects immersed in cold water. (NMRI)

- Report No. 1 - PROTECTIVE CLOTHING FOR SUBJECTS IMMERSED IN COLD WATER: PROTECTIVE VALUE OF WATER-TIGHT SUITS, 10 July 1943. (Newburgh and Spealman)

- Report No. 2 - PROTECTIVE CLOTHING FOR SUBJECTS IMMERSED IN COLD WATER. PART A. SOME CHARACTERISTICS OF THE "PASKE" SUIT (BRITISH CATAPULT SUIT). PART B. DEGREE OF PROTECTION AGAINST EVAPORATIVE COOLING AFFORDED BY WATERTIGHT SUITS, 10 August 1943. (Newburgh and Spealman)

- Report No. 3 - BODY COOLING OF MEN AND ANIMALS IMMERSED IN WATER, 5 February 1945. (Spealman)

- Report No. 4 - BODY COOLING IN WATER AND EFFECTIVENESS OF PETROLATUM IN RETARDING HEAT LOSS, 24 May 1945. (Spealman)

- Report No. 5 - REPORT ON CAPTURED ENEMY EQUIPMENT (CEE #6766, GERMAN FLYER'S IMMERSION SUIT), 24 July 1945. (Spealman and Catchpole)

- Report No. 6 - DESIGN AND CONSTRUCTION OF A CONTINUOUS WEAR EXPOSURE SUIT FOR THE BUREAU OF AERONAUTICS, 30 July 1945. (Margolis)

- Report No. 7 - EVALUATION OF BUAER AND ARMY QUICK DONNING EXPOSURE SUITS, 8 August 1945. (Spealman)

- Report No. 8 - A RATIONAL METHOD FOR DETERMINING LOCAL AND OVER-ALL INSULATION OF LOW TEMPERATURE CLOTHING, 19 September 1945. (Yaglou)

- Report No. 9 - COMPARATIVE COMFORT OF THE COMBINATION RAIN SUIT-EXPOSURE SUIT (RED STAR RUBBER COMPANY) AND NAVY PARKA RAIN CLOTHING, 29 October 1945. (Spealman and Margolis)

3. X-227 - Effectiveness and practicability of body armor in preventing injuries from bullets and other missiles. (NMRI)

- Report No. 4 - DESIGN OF ARMOR JACKET FOR AVIATION PERSONNEL, 5 October 1945. (Margolis and Shelesnyak)

4. X-373 - A study of the flash-resistant properties of flight clothing. (NMRI)

- Report - THE FLASH-RESISTANT PROPERTIES OF FABRICS PROPOSED FOR FLIGHT CLOTHING, 17 April 1944. (Fauley and Hyslop)

5. X-639 TED NAM 2596 - Winter flight clothing - automatic temperature control for. (NAES, Philadelphia)

- Report 2596.1 - GENERAL ELECTRIC CO. ELECTRICALLY HEATED FLIGHT SUITS - TYPES F3, F6, F4, FC1, and F5, 14 May 1945.

- Report 2596.1 - PART I - GENERAL ELECTRIC CO. AUTOMATIC TEMPERATURE CONTROL, CAT. NO. PX3A4, 14 July 1945. (Thomas)

- Report 2596.1 - PART II - TEST OF COLVINEX. ELECTRICALLY-HEATED FLIGHT SUIT, DESIGNED FOR -90°F., 17 August 1945. (Thomas)

6. X-640 - Body armor and wound ballistics. (Biodynamics Branch, Research Division, BUMED)

- Status Report - DIPHASIC ARMOR - 1. GLASS - DORON, 21 July 1945. (Webster)

- This work is summarized in the article, "DEVELOPMENT OF BODY ARMOR", October 1945. The Hospital Corps Quarterly, Vol. 18. (Webster)

7. X-711 TED NAM 25704 - Composite flight suit - development of. (NAES, Philadelphia) (No report, work continuing)

C. DENTISTRY

1. X-91 - Effect of aviation conditions on dental pulp and periosteum. (NMRI)

   - Report No. 1 - Same title as above, 24 June 1944. (Restarski and Gersh)

   - Report No. 2 - EFFECT OF AVIATION CONDITIONS ON THE DENTAL PULP AND PERIOSTEUM. II. VIBRATION, 20 October 1944. (Restarski)

2. X-157 - Study of Methods of Equalizing Middle Ear Pressure. (Pensacola)

   - Report - RELATIONSHIP OF DENTAL MALOCCLUSION TO EAR BLOCK IN THE LOW PRESSURE CHAMBER, 16 March 1943. (Brickman and Bierman)

3. X-355 - Dental reaction to high altitude environment. (Jacksonville)

   - Preliminary Report - Same title as above, July 1944. (Bunch and Beaton)

   - Final Report entitled as above, March 1945. (Bunch and Beaton)

4. X-587 - A study of aerodontalgia occurring during routine oxygen indoctrination in the low pressure chamber with a view to evolving a theory regarding its cause. (Quantico)

   - Report - Same title as above, 23 July 1945. (Hutchins, Reynolds, Werner and Philbrook)

5. X-604 - Evaluation of low pressure chamber as a diagnostic aid in dentistry. (NMRI and Naval Dental School) (No report, work continuing)

D. EAR NOSE AND THROAT

1. X-152 - Effect of nasal ventilation upon tubal-equalizing efficiency in flying personnel. (AOTC, Jacksonville)

- Report - Same title as above, October 1943. (MacGreagor and Sternstein)

- Final Report - EVALUATION OF THE NASAL RESISTANCE INHALER, A DEVICE FOR THE PREVENTION OF AERO-OTITIS AND AERO-SINUSITIS DEVISED BY LT. COMDR. H. J. STERNSTEIN (MC) USNR, 6 March 1945. (Carter and Beaton.

2. X-158 - Relationship of middle ear pressure to hearing in aviation. (Pensacola)

- Report - Same title as above, undated, no author given. (School of Aviation Medicine)

3. X-685 - Evaluation of use of nose clips to aid in equalization of the middle ear pressure of aviation personnel. (COMFAIR, Quonset) (No report, work continuing)

E. FOOD AND WATER

1. X-169 - Vitamin content of naval flight rations as affected by their method of cooking. (NMRI)

   - Report No. 1 - Same title as above, 16 October 1943. (Eakin and Gerard)

   - Report No. 2 - NUTRITIONAL AND BACTERIOLOGICAL EVALUATION OF THE MAXSON SKY PLATE, 25 August 1945. (Haugen, Sullivan and Duggan)

   - Report No. 3 - BACTERIOLOGICAL EXAMINATION OF MAXSON SKY PLATES SUBMITTED BY COMNATS, 11 January 1946, 4 April 1946. (Comploier and Gillmore)

2. X-280 TED UNL 2569 - Tests of self-heating food cans. (NMRI)

   - Report - Same title, 24 January 1944. (Pine)

3. X-316 - Self-selection of specific dietaries to satisfy nutritional requirements. (NMRI)

   - Report No. 1 - SELF SELECTION OF DIETS IN RATS RENDERED ANOXIC BY DECOMPRESSION TO ALTITUDE: I. SALT APPETITE, 27 November 1945. (Catchpole and Pine)

F. MOTION SICKNESS

1. X-72 - Motion Sickness. (Pensacola)

   - Report - THE INCIDENCE OF AIRSICKNESS AMONG AVIATION CADETS IN PATROL AIRCRAFT, April 1943. (School of Aviation Medicine)

2. X-252 - The effect of hyoscine on motion sickness in aircraft. (Pensacola)

   - Report No. 1 - Same title as above, 1 May 1944. (Lilienthal)

   - Report No. 2 - THE EFFECT OF HYOSCINE ON MOTION SICKNESS IN AIRCRAFT: INDIVIDUAL THERAPY OF MOTION SUSCEPTIBLE SUBJECTS, 2 March 1945. (Lilienthal)

3. X-278 - Motion sickness, validation of motion machines and procedures for the study of motion sickness, and the evaluation of motion sickness preventative. (NMRI)

   - Report No. 1 - SIDE EFFECTS OF THREE MOTION SICKNESS PREVENTIVES, 26 June 1944. (Birren, Stormont and Fisher)

   - Report No. 2 - AN EVALUATION OF A MOTION SICKNESS QUESTIONNAIRE IN PREDICTING SUSCEPTIBILITY TO SEA-SICKNESS, 15 August 1944. (Birren, Fisher and Stormont)

   - Report No. 3 - AN EVALUATION OF THE POTENTIALITY OF BULBOCAPNINE AS A MOTION SICKNESS PREVENTIVE, 16 August 1944. (Birren, Stormont and Pfeiffer)

   - Report No. 4 - REACTIONS TO NEOSTIGMINE AND APOMORPHINE AS INDICATION OF SUSCEPTIBILITY TO SEASICKNESS, 26 February 1945. (Birren, Stormont, and Pfeiffer)

   - Report No. 5 - OBSERVATIONS ON MEN HIGHLY SUSCEPTIBLE TO SEASICKNESS WITH REMARKS ON PERIODIC MOTION OF SHIPS, 17 July 1945. (Birren and Morales)

   - Report No. 6 - FURTHER STUDIES ON THE PREDICTION OF SUSCEPTIBILITY TO SEASICKNESS BY A MOTION SICKNESS QUESTIONNAIRE, 8 October 1945. (Birren and Fisher)

G. NITROGEN

1. X-43 - Measurements of gaseous exchange in connection with aviation and deep sea diving by technique employing radioactive substances. (Experimental Diving Unit, Navy Yard, Washington, D. C., and NMRI)

- Report - RATE OF ABSORPTION OF RADIOACTIVE KRYPTON MEASURED IN DEEP SEA DIVERS, 29 July 1942. (Behnke and Morgan)

- Report No. 1 - MEASUREMENTS OF GASEOUS EXCHANGE IN CONNECTION WITH AVIATION AND DEEP SEA DIVING BY TECHNIQUES EMPLOYING RADIOACTIVE SUBSTANCES - I. ON THE THEORY OF BLOOD - TISSUE EXCHANGES OF INERT GASES, 8 May 1944. (Smith and Morales)

- Report No. 2 - MEASUREMENTS OF GASEOUS EXCHANGE IN CONNECTION WITH AVIATION AND DEEP SEA DIVING BY TECHNIQUES EMPLOYING RADIOACTIVE SUBSTANCES - II. CIRCULATION AND INERT GAS EXCHANGES AT THE LUNG, 29 July 1944. (Morales and Smith)

- Report No. 3 - THE QUANTITATIVE PHYSIOLOGICAL BASIS OF INERT GAS EXCHANGE: APPLICATIONS TO DECOMPRESSION SICKNESS, 18 July 1945. (Morales, Smith and Behnke)

- Report No. 4 - ON THE POSSIBLE DETERMINATION OF GROSS HUMAN BODY COMPOSITION BY THE USE OF RADIOACTIVE INERT GASES, 1 August 1945. (Morales and Smith)

2. X-114 - Value of preliminary oxygen inhalation for prevention of decompression sickness during high altitude flight. (Experimental Diving Unit, Navy Yard, Washington, D. C.)

- Report - Same title as above, 15 December 1942. (Behnke, Welham and Yarbrough)

- Report - PRE-OXYGENATION IN THE PREVENTION OF BENDS; REST vs. EXERCISE, April 1943. (No author given)

3. X-141 - Effect of preoxygenation on aeroembolism. (Pensacola)

- Report - EFFECT OF PREOXYGENATION ON RESISTANCE TO AEROEMBOLISM: PREOXYGENATION IN SUSCEPTIBLE INDIVIDUALS, 16 February 1943. (Physiological Research Section and Oxygen Indoctrination Unit)

- Report - THE EFFECT OF PREOXYGENATION ON RESISTANCE TO DECOMPRESSION ILLNESS: STUDY FOR OPTIMAL TIME OF PREOXYGENATION, March 1943. (No author given)

4. X-201 - Influence of demand and air diluter demand oxygen systems used from sea level on the incidence of bends. (Pensacola)

- Report No. 1 - Same title as above, 2 November 1943. (McGoldrick, Lally and Langley)

5. X-284 - Determination of bubble formation in decompressed tissues by the measurement of specific gravity. Correlation of Bubble Formation in Susceptible Tissues with Vascularity and Fat Content. (NMRI)

- Report No. 1 - THE FORMATION AND APPEARANCE OF TISSUE AND VASCULAR GAS BUBBLES AFTER RAPID DECOMPRESSION OF GUINEA PIGS FROM HIGH PRESSURE ATMOSPHERES, 7 March 1944. (Gersh and Hawkinson)

- Report No. 2 - CHANGES IN SPECIFIC GRAVITY OF TISSUES, ORGANS, AND THE ANIMAL AS A WHOLE RESULTING FROM RAPID DECOMPRESSION OF GUINEA PIGS FROM HIGH PRESSURE ATMOSPHERES, 8 March 1944. (Gersh, Hawkinson, Rathbun and Behnke)

- Report No. 3 - RELATIONS OF CAPILLARIES TO FAT CELLS, 12 September 1944. (Gersh and Still)

- Report No. 4 - OBSERVATIONS OF GAS BUBBLES IN PIAL VESSELS OF CATS FOLLOWING RAPID DECOMPRESSION FROM HIGH PRESSURE ATMOSPHERES, 4 October 1944. (Wagner)

- Report No. 5 - COMPARISON OF VASCULAR AND EXTRA VASCULAR BUBBLES FOLLOWING DECOMPRESSION FROM HIGH PRESSURE ATMOSPHERES OF OXYGEN, HELIUM-OXYGEN, ARGON-OXYGEN AND AIR, 8 November 1944. (Gersh, Hawkinson, and Jenney)

- Report No. 6 - PHYSIOLOGICAL FACTORS AFFECTING THE PRODUCTION OF GAS BUBBLES IN RABBITS DECOMPRESSED TO ALTITUDE, 27 April 1945. (Catchpole and Gersh)

- Report No. 7 - BUBBLE FORMATION IN RABBITS DECOMPRESSED TO ALTITUDE: EFFECT OF PRE-OXYGENATION, ELECTRICAL STIMULATION, AND SOME PHARMACOLOGICAL FACTORS, 5 May 1945. (Catchpole and Gersh)

- Report No. 8 - APPEARANCE AND DISTRIBUTION OF GAS BUBBLES IN RABBITS DECOMPRESSED TO ALTITUDE, 7 May 1945. (Catchpole and Gersh)

- Report No. 9 - CORRELATION OF X-RAY AND GROSS OBSERVATIONS ON GAS BUBBLES IN GUINEA PIGS DECOMPRESSED FROM HIGH PRESSURE ATMOSPHERES, 9 May 1945. (Gersh)

- Report No. 10 - GAS BUBBLES IN BONE AND ASSOCIATED STRUCTURES, LUNG AND SPLEEN OF GUINEA PIGS DECOMPRESSED RAPIDLY FROM HIGH PRESSURE ATMOSPHERES, 10 May 1945. (Gersh)

6. X-338 - A procedure for selection of diving and aviation personnel resistant to decompression sickness based on tests in a low pressure chamber. (Experimental Diving Unit, Navy Yard, Washington, D. C.)

- Report No. 1 - Same title as above, January 1944. (Welham, Blanch and Behnke)

7. X-374 - Studies on factors affecting incidence of bends in low pressure chamber runs. (Miami)

- Report No. 1 - Same title as above, undated. (No author given)

- Report No. 2 - Same title as above, undated. (No author given)

- Report No. 3 - Same title as above, 27 July 1944. (Houston, Nuzie, Seitz and Besson)

8. X-609 - Decompression symptoms in low pressure chamber runs. (Pensacola)

- Report No. 1 - INCIDENCE TO BENDS PAIN IN A SHORT EXPOSURE TO SIMULATED ALTITUDES OF 26,000, 28,000, and 30,000 FEET, 1 September 1945. (Smedal and Brown)

H. ORIENTATION IN FLIGHT

1. X-148 - Disorientation in pilots. (Pensacola)

   - Report No. 1 - A PRELIMINARY REPORT ON STUDIES DEALING WITH THE AUTOKINETIC ILLUSION, 29 April 1944. (Graybiel and Clark)

   - Report No. 2 - THE EFFECT OF VARIOUS ARRANGEMENTS OF LIGHTS IN REDUCING AUTOKINESIS, 20 September 1944. (Graybiel, Clark and McNeal)

   - Report No. 3 - THE AUTOKINETIC ILLUSION AND ITS SIGNIFICANCE IN NIGHT FLYING, 7 February 1945. (Graybiel and Clark)

   - Report No. 4 - THE OCULO-GYRAL ILLUSION: A FORM OF APPARENT MOTION WHICH MAY BE OBSERVED FOLLOWING STIMULATION OF THE SEMICIRCULAR CANALS, 1 November 1945. (Graybiel and Hupp)

   - Report No. 5 - THE ROLE OF VESTIBULAR NYSTAGMUS IN THE VISUAL PERCEPTION OF A MOVING TARGET IN THE DARK, 14 January 1946. (Graybiel, Clark, MacCorquodale and Hupp)

   - Report No. 6 - THE ILLUSORY PERCEPTION OF MOVEMENT CAUSED BY ANGULAR ACCELERATION AND BY CENTRIFUGAL FORCE DURING FLIGHT. I. METHODOLOGY AND PRELIMINARY RESULTS, 25 March 1946. (Graybiel, Clark, and MacCorquodale)

   - Report No. 7 - THE CONCEPT OF AVIATOR'S "VERTIGO", 8 May 1946. (Vinacke)

   - Report No. 8 - THE ILLUSORY PERCEPTION OF MOVEMENT CAUSED BY ANGULAR ACCELERATION AND BY CENTRIFUGAL FORCE DURING FLIGHT. II. VISUALLY PERCEIVED MOVEMENT OF A FIXED TARGET DURING TURNS, 16 May 1946. (Clark, Graybiel and MacCorquodale)

   - Report No. 9 - ILLUSIONS EXPERIENCED BY AIRCRAFT PILOTS WHILE FLYING, 31 May 1946. (Vinacke)

2. X-259 - Disorientation of pilots in night and instrument flying, study of. (Anacostia)

   - Report - REPORT ON NIGHT FLYING DISORIENTATION, July 1944. (Beals and Luykx)

I. OXYGEN

Anoxia, Demonstration of

1. X-10 - Development of standardized procedures for the measurement of altitude tolerance. (Pensacola)

   - Report - PROGRESS REPORT OF RESEARCH, NAVAL AIR STATION, PENSACOLA, FLORIDA: AVIATION MEDICINE, RESEARCH PROJECT R7-1.11, May 1942. (No author given)

   - Report in letter form - WICKERS" PSYCHOMOTOR APPARATUS, 26 October 1942. (Buracker)

   - Report - PULSE RATES DURING ALTITUDE INDOCTRINATION RUNS, November 1942. (No author given)

   - Report - FINAL REPORT ON DOTTING APPARATUS AS A TEST OF ANOXIA, November 1942. (No author given)

   - Report - Second Report - THE EFFECT OF SULFATHIAZOLE UPON "ALTITUDE TOLERANCE" DETERMINED BY FLICKER FUSION TESTS, January 1943. (No author given)

   - Report - A STUDY OF BLOOD TYPES AND THEIR POSSIBLE RELATIONSHIP TO THE INCIDENCE OF DECOMPRESSION ILLNESS, July 1943. (Bierman)

   - Report - THE RELATIONSHIP OF AGE TO THE INCIDENCE OF DECOMPRESSION ILLNESS IN AVIATION, July 1943. (Bierman)

2. X-32 - Flicker fusion apparatus as a test of altitude tolerance. (Pensacola)

   - Report - PROGRESS REPORT OF RESEARCH, NAVAL AIR STATION, PENSACOLA, FLORIDA, 15 June 1942. (No author given)

   - Memorandum report - THE EFFECT OF ALTITUDE ON FLICKER FUSION, 21 August 1942. (No author given)

   - Report - FLICKER FUSION APPARATUS (ELECTRONIC OSCILLOSCOPE) AS A TEST OF "ALTITUDE TOLERANCE", November 1942. (No author given)

3. X-111 - Direct comparison of flicker fusion and dotter tests under comparative conditions of anoxia. (Pensacola)

- Report - THE EFFECT OF ACUTE ANOXIA UPON FLICKER, DOTTING AND HAND-WRITING TESTS IN TWENTY UNTRAINED SUBJECTS, 10 November 1942. (School of Aviation Medicine)

4. X-153 - Influence of anoxia on contract discrimination. (Pensacola)

- Report - INFLUENCE OF ANOXIA ON VISUAL CONTRACT DISCRIMINATION, 18 March 1943. (Hecht and Peckham)

- Preliminary Report - LOSS OF VISUAL CONTRACT DISCRIMINATION DURING ANOXIA, 4 June 1943. (No author given)

5. X-159 - Simplified flicker fusion apparatus applied as a test of altitude tolerance. (NMRI)

- Report - THE DESIGN AND CONSTRUCTION OF A SIMPLIFIED ELECTRONIC FLICKER-FUSION APPARATUS AND THE DETERMINATION OF ITS EFFECTIVENESS IN DETECTING ANOXIA, 1 December 1943. (Draeger and Fauley)

6. X-282 - Development of a test to demonstrate the effects of anoxia on flight personnel. (Seattle)

- Final Report - A NEW TEST FOR DEMONSTRATING THE EFFECTS OF MILDER DEGREES OF ANOXIA, 12 February 1946. (Gerstell)

7. X-283 - Development of a test to demonstrate the effects of anoxia on flight personnel. (Pensacola)

- Report No. 1 - CARD SORTING TEST FOR DEMONSTRATION OF ANOXIA. SOME FACTORS INFLUENCING SCORES MADE ON THE SEATTLE CARD SORTING TESTS, 3 June 1944. (West, Brown, James and Burt)

8. X-431 - Development of anoxia demonstration procedure for altitude training units on basis of breath holding ability. (Pensacola)

- Report No. 1 - BREATH HOLDING AT ALTITUDE AND BREATH HOLDING AS A DEMONSTRATION OF ANOXIA: PART I. BREATH HOLDING ABILITY AT ALTITUDE. PART II. BREATH HOLDING AS A DEMONSTRATION OF ANOXIA, 5 October 1944. (Brown)

9. X-538 - An investigation of the effect of altitude on night vision. (Alameda)

- Report No. 1 - Same title as above, 1 June 1945. (Price and Fuller)

10. X-564 - M-N Device for testing and demonstrating night vision under anoxic conditions. (Vero Beach)

- Report No. 1 - (Final) - A REPORT ON THE M-N DEVICE FOR DEMONSTRATING ANOXIC EFFECTS ON NIGHT VISION AND DAY VISION, 10 September 1945. (Moore, Nuzie and Sonn)

11. X-580 - Low pressure chamber demonstration of the effect of anoxia on night vision. (ComFair, Quonset Point and NAS, Grosse Ile., Michigan)

- Report No. 1 - A SIMPLE DEVICE FOR DEMONSTRATING THE EFFECT OF ANOXIA UPON SCOTOPIC VISION AT ALTITUDES BELOW 18,000 FEET, 9 May 1945. (Grinsted)

- Memorandum Report - A DEMONSTRATION OF THE EFFECTS OF ANOXIA UPON SCOTOPIC VISION, 22 May 1945. (Maynard, this report is regarded as Report No. 2)

- Report No. 3 - LOW PRESSURE CHAMBER DEMONSTRATION OF THE EFFECT OF ANOXIA ON NIGHT VISION HELD AT NAS, GROSSE ILE, MICHIGAN, 28 November 1945, 12 December 1945. (No author given)

12. X-593 - Measurement and demonstration of loss of visual function associated with anoxia. (Miami)

- Report No. 1 - THE EFFECT OF ANOXIA ON NIGHT VISION, 18 September 1945. (Seitz)

- Report No. 2 - SUBJECTIVE CHANGES IN ILLUMINATION WHEN OXYGEN IS USED FOLLOWING A PERIOD OF ANOXIA, 5 November 1945. (Seitz, Young, Besson, Evans and Hopkins)

13. X-667 - Evaluation of Quonset Anoxia Demonstration Device. (Pensacola)

- Report No. 1 - Same title as above, 25 January 1946. (Smedal, Hoffman, Brown and Daugherty)

OXYGEN

Equipment

1. X-85 - Effect of increased expiratory pressure in demand oxygen systems. (Pensacola)

- Preliminary Report - PRELIMINARY REPORT OF EXPIRATORY RESISTANCE MASK OBTAINED FROM OXYGEN EQUIPMENT COMPANY, NEW YORK, N. Y., December 1942. (No author given)

- Final Report - EFFECTS OF INCREASED EXPIRATORY PRESSURE IN DEMAND OXYGEN SYSTEMS, 18 February 1943. (No author given)

2. X-119 - (1) Design, modification and testing of oxygen breathing equipment, and (2) study of absorbent for the removal of carbon dioxide and water in oxygen breathing equipment. (NMRI)

- Report No. 1 - TESTS ON RINSING AND PERFORMANCE AT LOW TEMPERATURES OF THE F. W. B. RECIRCULATOR, 29 September 1943. (White and King)

3. X-143 - Comparative testing of British, Canadian, U. S. Army and Navy oxygen equipment. (Pensacola)

- Report No. 1 - COMPARATIVE TESTING OF OXYGEN EQUIPMENT. RETEST OF A-14 DEMAND OXYGEN MASKS., 23 September 1943. (Gemmill, Steele, Bierman, and Riley)

- Report No. 2 - COMPARATIVE TESTING OF OXYGEN EQUIPMENT, 21 January 1944. (Gemmill and Fugitt)

- Report - IMPROVEMENTS OF TYPE D MASK - MINE SAFETY APPLIANCES COMPANY. (Undated) (School of Aviation Medicine)

- Report - SUMMARY OF RESEARCH - COMPARATIVE TESTING OF OXYGEN EQUIPMENT. (Undated) (School of Aviation Medicine)

4. X-174 - Comparative Oxygen Economy of Oxygen Equipment. (Pensacola)

- Report No. 1 - (Preliminary) - DETERMINATION OF

- COMPARATIVE OXYGEN ECONOMIES OF OXYGEN EQUIPMENT, 1 October 1943. (Gemmill and Riley)

- Report No. 2 - DETERMINATION OF COMPARATIVE OXYGEN ECONOMIES OF OXYGEN EQUIPMENT, 6 December 1943. (Gemmill and Riley)

- Report No. 3 - DETERMINATION OF COMPARATIVE OXYGEN ECONOMIES OF OXYGEN EQUIPMENT: ECONOMIES OF CANADIAN DILUTER DEMAND, GERMAN DILUTER DEMAND AND U. S. ARMY PRESSURE DEMAND REGULATORS, 20 March 1944. (Weatherby)

- Report No. 4 - DETERMINATION OF COMPARATIVE OXYGEN ECONOMIES OF OXYGEN EQUIPMENT: PHYSIOLOGICAL TESTING OF ENGLISH (RAF) MASK, TYPE H, 13 January 1944. (Gemmill and Fugitt)

5. X-216 - Study of British bail-out oxygen equipment. (NMRI)

- Report No. 1 - Same title as above, 11 November 1943. (King, Futcher, and Pecora)

6. X-239 TED PTR 2516 - Physiological studies and test of oxygen and miscellaneous flight equipment at high altitudes under actual flight conditions. (Patuxent and NMRI)

- Report No. 1 - FLIGHT TESTS ON OXYGEN SYSTEMS FOR TRANSPORT PLANES AND ADDITIONAL PHYSIOLOGICAL OBSERVATIONS ON FLIGHT FROM PATUXENT RIVER, MARYLAND TO PORT LYAUTEY, NORTH AFRICA, 21 June 1944. (Weaver and King)

7. X-241 - Temperature indicating ink for demonstration of activity of MSA rebreather canister. (NAS, San Diego)

- Report - (Letter) - A NEW METHOD FOR APPRAISING THE OVERALL EFFICIENCY OF THE MSA REBREATHER, 23 September 1943. (Jones)

- Supplementary Report, November 1943. (No author given)

8. X-248 - Tests of Oxygen Masks MRS-1. (NMRI)

- Report - (Preliminary) - EXAMINATION OF EXPERIMENTAL SUSPENSION FOR THE MRS-1 OXYGEN MASK, 16 November 1943. (King)

- Report No. 1 - APPRAISAL OF THE SUSPENSION AND FIT OF THE MRS-1 OXYGEN MASK, 5 September 1944. (Henson and King)

9. X-249 TED UNL 2534 - Test of MSA Rebreather Employing Experimental Models of Pump Type Autovent Devices. (NMRI)

- Report - PHYSIOLOGICAL APPRAISAL OF MSA REBREATHER EMPLOYING EXPERIMENTAL MODELS OF PUMP TYPE AUTOVENT DEVICES: TYPE II AND III D, 4 February 1944. (Shelesnyak and Whaley)

10. X-251 - Respiratory metabolism of pilots and crew in planes. (Pensacola)

- Report No. 1 - RESPIRATORY METABOLISM OF PILOTS AND CREW IN PLANES.
  Sub-titles: 1. RESPIRATORY ACTIVITY OF MACHINE GUNNERS AT SEA LEVEL.
  2. DETERMINATION OF PEAK FLOWS OF OXYGEN EQUIPMENT.
  3. RELATIONSHIP OF RESPIRATORY MINUTE VOLUME TO OXYGEN CONSUMPTION UNDER CONDITIONS OF WORK, ANOXIA AND COLD.
  20 February 1944. (Gemmill, Weatherby, Lilienthal, and Riley)

11. X-257 - Tests of British Oxygen Mask Type "H". (NMRI)

- Report - PHYSIOLOGICAL APPRAISAL OF THE BRITISH OXYGEN MASK, TYPE "H", 6 January 1944. (NMRI) (King, Henson, and Whaley) Also published as CAM Report No. 281, 6 January 1944.

12. X-272 - Physiological tests of the A-10A Oxygen Masks. (Pensacola)

- Report No. 1 - PHYSIOLOGICAL TESTING OF A-10A OXYGEN MASKS, 13 January 1944. (Gemmill and Fugitt)

13. X-273 TED UNL 2553 - Physiological testing of the A-10A oxygen masks. (NMRI)

- Report - PHYSIOLOGICAL APPRAISAL OF A-10A OXYGEN MASK, 29 December 1943. (King, Futcher, Henson, and Whaley)

14. X-275 - Physiological testing of MSA type E experimental oxygen mask. (NMRI)

- Report - (Preliminary) - PHYSIOLOGICAL APPRAISAL OF THE MSA, TYPE E UNLINED EXPERIMENTAL OXYGEN MASK, 31 December 1943. (Henson, Whaley and King)

15. X-277 - Physiological testing of MSA type E experimental Oxygen Mask. (Pensacola)

- Report No. 1 - PHYSIOLOGICAL TESTING OF MSA TYPE E EXPERIMENTAL OXYGEN MASK, 7 January 1944. (Gemmill and Fugitt)

- Appendix A to Report No. 1 bearing the same title as Report No. 1, 25 February 1944. (Gemmill and Fugitt)

16. X-305 - Inspiratory resistances of the diluter demand regulator. (Cherry Point)

- Report No. 1 - (Final and Supplement) - INSPIRATORY RESISTANCES IN THE MASK WITH THE USE OF THE PIONEER DILUTER-DEMAND AND THE ARO-A 12 REGULATORS, 4 April 1944. (Eckman)

17. X-314 TED UNL 2579 - Physiological evaluation of Baldwin Rubber Company mask. (Pensacola)

- Report No. 1 - (Final) - PHYSIOLOGICAL TESTING OF BALDWIN RUBBER COMPANY MASK, 5 April 1944. (Gemmill and Fugitt)

18. X-315 - Use of Pioneer Diluter Demand Regulator by two individuals. (Seattle)

- Report - TWO MEN CAN USE ONE DILUTER DEMAND OXYGEN REGULATOR (PIONEER), January 1944.

- Report - EMERGENCY USE OF THE DILUTER DEMAND OXYGEN REGULATOR (PIONEER) BY TWO MEN. THIS REPORT WAS SUBMITTED BY NMRI AND KNOWN AS NMRI-55, 16 March 1944. (King and Shelesnyak)

19. X-320 - The percent distribution of the three sizes of Army A-14 masks required by naval aviators and air crewmen. (Norfolk)

- Report - THE PERCENT DISTRIBUTION OF THE THREE SIZES OF ARMY A-14 MASKS REQUIRED BY NAVAL AVIATORS AND AIR CREWMEN, 20 April 1944. (James, Poel, Dury, and Swearingen)

20. X-324

- Peak rates of oxygen flow from oxygen supply systems. (Pensacola)
- Report No. 1 - PEAK RATES OF OXYGEN FLOW FROM OXYGEN SUPPLY SYSTEMS, 26 June 1944. (Weatherby and Burt)
- Report No. 2 - PEAK RATES OF OXYGEN FLOW FROM OXYGEN SUPPLY SYSTEMS: DESCRIPTION OF A LOW INERTIA FLOW-METER, 13 December 1944. (Weatherby and Burt)
- Report No. 3 - PEAK RATES OF OXYGEN FLOW FROM OXYGEN SUPPLY SYSTEMS, 1 March 1945. (Weatherby and Burt)
- Report No. 4 - PEAK RATES OF OXYGEN FLOW FROM OXYGEN SUPPLY SYSTEMS: EFFECT OF SURGE TANKS ON PEAK RATES, 5 March 1945. (Weatherby and Burt)
- Report No. 5 - PEAK RATES OF OXYGEN FLOW FROM OXYGEN SUPPLY SYSTEMS: FREQUENCY OF SIMULTANEOUS INSPIRATIONS IN A GROUP OF TEN SUBJECTS, 12 April 1945. (Weatherby and Burt)
- Report No. 6 - PEAK RATES OF OXYGEN FLOW FROM OXYGEN SUPPLY SYSTEMS: INFLUENCE OF A SURGE TANK ON A SYSTEM SUPPLIED BY LIQUID OXYGEN CONVERTERS, 30 April 1945. (Weatherby)
- Report No. 7 - PEAK RATES OF OXYGEN FLOW FROM OXYGEN SUPPLY SYSTEMS: MASK SUCTION AND SENSATIONS OBSERVED DURING RESTRICTION OF INSPIRATORY FLOW, 30 May 1945. (Weatherby)
- Letter report - SUMMARY OF FINDINGS INCLUDED IN REPORTS NOS. 1, 3, 5, and 7, 13 June 1945. (Iverson)

21. X-344

- Physiological test of MRS-1 oxygen mask. (Pensacola)
- Report No. 1 - (Final) - PHYSIOLOGICAL TESTING OF MRS-1 OXYGEN MASK, 26 March 1944. (Gemmill and Fugitt)
- Preliminary Report: Appendix A. - ACOUSTICAL EVALU-ATION: COMPARATIVE TESTING OF EXPERIMENTAL OXYGEN

- MASKS, 12 April 1944. (Steer and Lawrence)

22. X-353 TED UNL 2587 - Physiological testing of NDRC full face experimental oxygen mask. (Pensacola)

- Report No. 1 - (Final) - PHYSIOLOGICAL TESTING OF NDRC FULL FACE EXPERIMENTAL OXYGEN MASK, 1 May 1944. (Gemmill and ugitt)

23. X-363 - Leakage in the A-10A Mask, as determined by the McKesson Leak Test. (San Diego)

- Report No. 1 - (Final) - LEAKAGE IN THE ACUSHNET A-10A OXYGEN FACE MASK AS DETERMINED BY THE McKESSON LEAK TESTER, April 1944. (Mueller, Pope, Vollmer, Walker, and Sharpe)

24. X-387 - Evaluation of Canadian mask size templates for possible use in fitting A-14 oxygen masks. (Pensacola)

- Report No. 1 - (Final) - EVALUATION OF CANADIAN MASK SIZE TEMPLATE FOR POSSIBLE USE IN FITTING A-14 OXYGEN MASKS, 6 May 1944. (Gemmill and Fugitt)

25. X-391 TED UNL 2592 - Physiological evaluation of available continuous flow oxygen apparatus from the point of view of use in Navy transport planes. (NMRI and Patuxent)

- Report - Preliminary Data - Same title as above, 23 May 1944. (Goldman, Shelesnyak, and King) (Designated as Report No. 1)

- Report No. 2 - EVALUATION OF CONSTANT FLOW-RESERVOIR OXYGEN MASK SYSTEM FOR USE IN NAVY TRANSPORT PLANES, 1 August 1944. (Goldman)

26. X-397 - Determination of relative proportion of three sizes of A-14 oxygen mask required by naval personnel. (Cherry Point)

- Report No. 1 - DETERMINATION OF RELATIVE PROPORTIONS OF THREE SIZES OF A-14 OXYGEN MASKS REQUIRED BY NAVAL PERSONNEL, 17 June 1944. (Borofsky, Eckman, and Renaud)

27. X-405 - Inspiratory resistance of Pioneer diluter demand regulator with diluter "on" in presence of failure of oxygen supply. (Cherry Point)

- Report No. 1 - SUBJECTIVE REACTIONS AND INSPIRATORY RESISTANCES OF PIONEER DILUTER-DEMAND REGULATOR WITH DILUTER "ON" IN PRESENCE OF FAILURE OF OXYGEN SUPPLY, 31 July 1944. (Borofsky and Renaud)

28. X-415 - Fabrication of a light helmet for oxygen inhalation. (NMRI)

- Report No. 1 - AN IMPROVED HELMET FOR BREATHING OXYGEN OR OTHER GASES, 30 December 1945. (Duncan)

29. X-438 TED UNL 25113 - Determination of degree of inspiratory resistance which will warn of failure of oxygen supply to diluter demand regulator. (Pensacola)

- Report No. 1 - (Final) - DETERMINATION OF DEGREE OF INSPIRATORY RESISTANCE WHICH WILL WARN OF FAILURE OF OXYGEN SUPPLY TO DILUTER DEMAND REGULATOR, 30 September 1944. (Weatherby)

30. X-440 TED UNL 25119 - Physiological evaluation of U. S. Army H-2 bail-out oxygen equipment. (NMRI)

- Report - PHYSIOLOGICAL EVALUATION OF U. S. ARMY AIR FORCES H-2 BAIL-OUT OXYGEN EQUIPMENT, 28 August 1944. (Shelesnyak, Whaley, and Goldman)

31. X-459 - Simulated Service testing of DJ-1 Oxygen Flow Indicator and Comparison with other indicators. (San Diego)

- Report - SIMULATED SERVICE TESTING OF DJ-1 OXYGEN FLOW INDICATOR AND COMPARISON WITH OTHER INDICATORS, August 1944. (No author given)

32. X-478 - Simulated Service testing of DJ-2 oxygen flow indicators and comparison with DJ-1 oxygen flow indicators. (San Diego)

- Report - SIMULATED SERVICE TEST OF DJ-2 OXYGEN FLOW INDICATORS AND COMPARISON WITH OTHER INDICATORS. (Undated) (No author given)

33. X-481 - Development of a pressure and flow recorder for laboratory and field studies of respiration and of breathing equipment. (NMRI)

- No report. Work continuing.

34. X-485 - An evaluation of the A-14 oxygen demand mask. (San Diego)

- Report No. 1 - (Final) - AN EVALUATION OF THE A-14 OXYGEN DEMAND MASK. (Undated) (Mueller, Pope, Sharpe, Sweeney, Barrington, Yarbrough, Baur, and Ballentine)

35. X-508 - Oxygen accumulation within altitude chambers. (Miami)

- Report No. 1 - A METHOD FOR DETERMINING OXYGEN ACCUMULATION IN ALTITUDE CHAMBER DURING ROUTINE INDOCTRINATION RUNS, 5 December 1944. (Altitude Training Unit Staff)

- Letter Report to Capt. J. H. Korb (MC) USN from Capt. A. B. Chesser (MC) USN, 9 August 1945.

36. X-512 - Evaluation of standard male quick disconnect fitting for oxygen line modified to give warning of accidental detachment. (Pensacola)

- Report No. 1 - EVALUATION OF STANDARD MALE QUICK DISCONNECT FITTING FOR OXYGEN LINE MODIFIED TO GIVE WARNING OF ACCIDENTAL DETACHMENT, 20 January 1945. (Weatherby and Burt)

37. X-525 - Test of mask fit during movement and in the cold. (Pensacola)

- Report No. 1 - TEST OF MASK FIT DURING MOVEMENT AND IN THE COLD, 15 March 1945. (Riley and Fugitt)

38. X-551 TED UNL 25173 - Physiological evaluation of diluter demand oxygen regulators with safety pressure. (NMRI)

- Report No. 1 - PHYSIOLOGICAL EVALUATION OF THREE PIONEER BENDIX DILUTER DEMAND OXYGEN REGULATORS WITH SAFETY PRESSURE, 13 April 1945. (Goldman, King, Henson, Vollmer, Whaley, and Perkins)

- Report No. 2 - OXYGEN EXPENDITURE OF SAFETY PRESSURE DILUTER DEMAND OXYGEN REGULATORS, 14 December 1945. (Goldman, Vollmer, and Henson)

39. X-569 - Physiological testing of three sizes of improved NDRC full face Type A-16 experimental oxygen mask. (Pensacola)

- Report No. 1 - PHYSIOLOGICAL TESTING OF THREE SIZES OF IMPROVED NDRC FULL FACE TYPE A-16 EXPERIMENTAL OXYGEN MASK, 8 June 1945. (Fugitt)

40. X-584 TED UNL 25186 - Evaluation of certain characteristics of the type A-14 oxygen mask with baffles over the mask inlet ports. (Pensaco a)

- Report No. 1 - EVALUATION OF CERTAIN CHARACTERISTICS OF THE TYPE A-14 OXYGEN MASK WITH BAFFLES OVER THE MASK INLET PORTS, 13 August 1945. (White) This report covers TED UNL 25186.1.

41. X-592 TED UNL 25196 - Evaluation of Acushnet Process Company oxygen mask for use in transport aircraft. (Pensacola)

- Report No. 1 - EVALUATION OF ACUSHNET PROCESS COMPANY OXYGEN MASK FOR USE IN TRANSPORT AIRCRAFT, 14 June 1945. (Fugitt and Riley)

42. X-597 TED UNL 25210 - An instrument for service testing diluter demand oxygen regulators in aircraft. (Pensacola)

- Report No. 1 - INSTRUMENT FOR SERVICE TESTING DILUTER-DEMAND OXYGEN EQUIPMENT IN AIRCRAFT: CONSTRUCTION USE AND EVALUATION, 6 November 1945. (Skow)

- Report No. 2 - INSTRUMENT FOR SERVICE TESTING DILUTER-DEMAND OXYGEN EQUIPMENT IN AIRCRAFT: TESTING PROCEDURE AND MAINTENANCE OF, 17 November 1945. (Skow) This report is designated as "Development Report... Airframe Accessories" #2-45.

43. X-600 - Analysis of the operating qualities of 480 Pioneer diluter demand oxygen regulators. (Pensacola)

- Report No. 1 - ANALYSIS OF THE OPERATING QUALITIES OF 480 PIONEER DILUTER DEMAND OXYGEN REGULATORS, 30 June 1945. (Malone)

44. X-601 TED UNL 25200 TED PEN 2502 - Preliminary evaluation of MSA Diluter Demand AN-R-5 regulators, Serial Nos. 45-64 and 45-67. (Pensacola)

- Report No. 1 - PRELIMINARY EVALUATION OF MSA DILUTER DEMAND AN-R-5 REGULATORS, SERIAL NOS. 45-64 and 45-67, 29 June 1945. (Malone)

- Report No. 1 in TED No. PEN 2502 - DETERMINATION OF OXYGEN EXPENDITURE OF TWO MSA DILUTER DEMAND AN-R-5 REGULATORS, Serial Nos. 45-64 and 45-67, 13 November 1945. (Malone)

45. X-611 - Determination of permissible expiratory resistances in aircraft oxygen equipment. (Pensacola)

- Report No. 1 - PERMISSIBLE EXPIRATORY RESISTANCES IN AIRCRAFT OXYGEN EQUIPMENT, 1 September 1945. (Weatherby)

46. X-623 TED UNL 25196 - Oxygen Masks, Type 14. (Pensacola)

- Report No. 1 - TED UNL 25196.1 - OXYGEN MASKS, TYPE A-14, SUSPENSION OF FROM FABRIC STRAP - EVALUATION OF, 27 June 1945. (Weatherby)

- Report No. 2 - TED UNL 25196.1 - OXYGEN MASKS, TYPE A-14, SUSPENSION OF FROM NAVY HEADSET - EVALUATION OF, 7 July 1945. (Author unknown)

47. X-625 TED PEN 2501 - Japanese aviation oxygen equipment-chemical oxygen generator - test of. (Pensacola)

- Report No. 1 - JAPANESE CHEMICAL OXYGEN GENERATOR, TEST OF, 1 August 1945. (Weatherby)

48. X-626 TED NAM 25508 - Aircraft oxygen cylinder valves - flow tests on. (Pensacola)

- Report - TED No. NAM 25508 - AIRCRAFT OXYGEN VALVES - TEST OF, 17 March 1945. (Hays and Cherry)

- Report - TED No. NAM 25508.2 - AIRCRAFT HIGH PRESSURE OXYGEN LINE VALVE - MANUFACTURED BY SUPERIOR VALVE AND FITTING COMPANY - QUALIFICATION TEST OF. (Date and Author unknown)

- Report - TED No. NAM 25508.3 - AIRCRAFT HIGH PRESSURE OXYGEN LINE VALVE - MANUFACTURED BY BASTIAN BLESSING COMPANY - QUALIFICATION TEST OF, 14 July 1945. (Hays)

- Report - TED No. NAM 25508.4 - AIRCRAFT OXYGEN CYLINDER VALVES, MANUFACTURED BY SUPERIOR VALVE AND FITTING

- COMPANY - QUALIFICATION TEST OF, 31 May 1945. (Hays)

- Report - TED No. NAM 25508.5 - AIRCRAFT OXYGEN CYLINDER VALVES - FLOW TESTS ON, 14 June 1945. (Hays)

- Report - TED No. NAM 25508.6 - AIRCRAFT HIGH PRESSURE OXYGEN LINE VALVE (TYPE 411) MANUFACTURED BY THE W. J. SCHOENBERGER COMPANY - QUALIFICATION TEST OF, 28 August 1945. (Hays)

- Report - TED No. NAM 25508.7 - AIRCFAFT HIGH OXYGEN CYLINDER VALVE (No. 5564) MANUFACTURED BY SUPERIOR VALVE AND FITTING COMPANY, - QUALIFICATION TEST OF, 14 July 1945. (Hays)

- Report - TED No. NAM 25508.8 - AIRCRAFT OXYGEN CYLINDER VALVES (TWO PIECE BODY DESIGN) MANUFACTURED BY SUPERIOR VALVE AND FITTING COMPANY, 5 January 1946. (Cherry)

- Report - TED No. NAM 25508.9 - AIRCRAFT OXYGEN CYLINDER VALVE MANUFACTURED BY KEROTEST MFG. COMPANY - QUALIFICATION TEST OF, 4 February 1946. (Cherry)

- Report - TED No. NAM 25508.10 - HIGH PRESSURE OXYGEN LINE VALVE (TYPE 8021) MFG. BY KEROTEST MFG. COMPANY QUALIFICATION TEST OF, 18 January 1946. (Cherry)

49. X-628 - Respiratory data for design of aircraft oxygen equipment - Determination of. (NIH)

- No report. Work continuing.

50. X-629 TED NAM 25742 - Oxygen cylinders, flexible shaft and casing combination for remote control of. (Philadelphia)

- Report - TED No. NAM 25742 - OXYGEN CYLINDERS FLEXIBLE SHAFT AND CASING COMBINATION FOR REMOTE CONTROL OF (S. S. WHITE DENTAL MFG. CO.) - EVALUATION OF, 27 January 1945. (Meakin)

- Report - TED No. NAM 25742.1 - REMOTE CONTROL OF OXYGEN CYLINDERS FLEXIBLE SHAFT AND CASING DEVICE - INVESTIGATION OF, 18 January 1946. (Meakin and Cherry)

51. X-637 TED UNL 25209 - Evaluation of use of fixed oxygen installations in escape from ditched aircraft. (NMRI)

- Report No. 1 - EVALUATION OF THE USE OF FIXED OXYGEN INSTALLATIONS IN SUBMERGED AIRCRAFT, 8 January 1946. (Duffner)

52. X-641 TED UNL 2591 - Moisture condensation in diluter demand oxygen regulators - determination of. (Pensacola)

- Report No. 1 - (Final) - MOISTURE CONDENSATION IN DILUTER DEMAND OXYGEN REGULATORS - DETERMINATION OF, 28 June 1944.
  Sub-titles: (a) FROSTING OF DILUTER DEMAND OXYGEN REGULATORS INSTALLED IN LOW PRESSURE CHAMBER. (Skow)
  (b) EXAMINATION OF DILUTER DEMAND OXYGEN REGULATORS USED IN THE SOUTH PACIFIC AREA. (Gemmill)

53. X-642 TED UNL 2593 - The connection and quick disconnect for adapting diluter demand oxygen regulator for use of two men. (Pensacola)

- Report No. 1 - TEE CONNECTION AND QUICK DISCONNECT FOR ADAPTING DILUTER DEMAND OXYGEN REGULATOR FOR USE OF TWO MEN -- TEST OF, 15 May 1944. (Weatherby)

54. X-643 TED UNL 2598 - Chest type diluter demand oxygen regulator. (Pensacola)

- Report No. 1 - TESTING OF THE CHEST TYPE DILUTER DEMAND OXYGEN REGULATOR MANUFACTURED BY ARO EQUIPMENT CORPORATION, 24 July 1944. (Fugitt)

- Report - CHEST TYPE DILUTER DEMAND OXYGEN REGULATOR - MANUFACTURED BY ARO EQUIPMENT CORPORATION - TEST OF, 20 April 1945. (Nisbet and Skow)

55. X-646 TED UNL 25181 - Helmets, flying oxygen mask attachment. (Pensacola)

- Report TED No. UNL 25181 - Untitled. 21 July 1945. (Skow, Schivley, Kellerman, and Rhoades)

- Work is continuing.

56. X-653 TED NAM 25525 - Low pressure portable diluter demand oxygen regulator. (Philadelphia)

- Report - TED NAM-25525 - A-14 MASK HEATERS, GENERAL ELECTRIC COMPANY, MODELS PG-6A3 and P-291-32, December 1944. (Thomas and Meakin)

- Report - TED NAM-25525.1 - DILUTER DEMAND OXYGEN EQUIPMENT REGULATOR - LOW INLET SUPPLY PRESSURE TYPE - TEST OF, 15 January 1945. (WIGGINS LABORATORY, CUYHAUGA FALLS, OHIO) (Watts and Wilson)

- Report - TED No. NAM 25525.2 - LOW PRESSURE PORTABLE DILUTER DEMAND OXYGEN REGULATOR MANUFACTURED BY ARO EQUIPMENT COMPANY - TEST OF, 27 July 1945. (Watts)

57. X-654 TED NAM 25671 - Oxygen regulators. (Philadelphia)

- Report - TED No. NAM 25671 - READY ROOM OXYGEN MASK LEAKAGE AND BREATHING TUBE QUICK DISCONNECT PULL APART TEST PANEL - DEVELOPMENT OF, 22 June 1945. (Meakin)

- Report - TED No. NAM 25671.1 - DILUTER DEMAND OXYGEN REGULATOR TESTER FOR TESTING IN AIRCRAFT - DEVELOPMENT OF, 7 June 1945. (Watts and Hays)

58. X-666 - The development of flow meters of low inertia and rapidity of response for use in connection with studies on respiratory exchange and distribution of oxygen. (Pensacola)

- No report. Work continuing.

59. X-668 TED NAM 25672 - Oxygen masks - test of. (Philadelphia)

- Report - TED No. NAM 25672 - OXYGEN MASK, TYPE A-14 - SUSPENSION FOR, TEST OF, 19 March 1945. (Hamilton)

- Report - TED No. NAM 25672.1 - OXYGEN MASK, TYPE A8B, TEST OF SUSPENSION FOR, 14 September 1945. (Thomas)

- Report - TED No. NAM 25672.2 - OXYGEN TRANSPORT MASK (ACUSHNET PROCESS CO.), 13 September 1945. (Thomas)

- Report - TED No. NAM 25672.3 - OXYGEN TRANSPORT MASK (MINE SAFETY APPLICANCE CO.) - TEST OF, 17 September 1945. (Perkinson, Jr.)

- Report - TED No. NAM 25672.4 - OXYGEN TRANSPORT MASK, MODEL XTA WITH ALTERED VALVE SHIELD (ACUSHNET

- PROCESS CO.) - TEST OF, 21 December 1945. (Hodapp)

60. X-679 - Practical test of methods for cleaning oxygen masks for transport aircraft and low pressure chambers. (Pensacola)

- Report No. 1 - A PRACTICAL METHOD FOR CLEANING THE A-14 TYPE OXYGEN MASK, 1 March 1946. (Smedal, Brown, Jr., Hoffman, and Daugherty)

61. X-681 TED NAM 25491 - Emergency oxygen bail-out equipment - development of. (Philadelphia)

- Report - TED NAM-25491 - EMERGENCY OXYGEN BAIL-OUT EQUIPMENT FOR ALTITUDES BELOW 40,000 FEET - DEVELOPMENT OF, 12 March 1945. (Hays and Watts)

- Report - TED No. NAM 25491.2 - POSITIVE PRESSURE BREATHING EQUIPMENT - WIND CURRENTS ON DURING BAIL-OUT - EFFECT OF, 18 October 1945. (Watts)

- Report - TED No. NAM 25491.3 - EMERGENCY BAIL-OUT EQUIPMENT FOR ALTITUDES BELOW 40,000 FEET - DEVELOPMENT OF, 3 April 1946. (Scott)

62. X-687 TED PTR 2516 - Flight tests of Pioneer-Bendix diluter demand oxygen regulator with safety pressure. (Patuxent River)

- Report - (Preliminary) - TED No. PTR 2516.1- FLIGHT TESTS OF PIONEER-BENDIX DILUTER DEMAND OXYGEN REGULATOR WITH SAFETY PRESSURE, 1 November 1945. (Eckman and Mathis)

63. X-688 TED NAM 25752 - Eclipse Pioneer diluter demand oxygen regulator with safety pressure - Test of. (Philadelphia)

- Letter Report - (Interim) - TED No. NAM 25752 - SUBJECT ECLIPSE PIONEER DILUTER-DEMAND OXYGEN REGULATOR WITH SAFETY PRESSURE - TEST OF: DISCUSSION OF THE IMPORATNCE OF THE SAFETY FACTOR AFFORDED BY SAFETY PRESSURE, 15 November 1945. (Scott)

- Report - TED NAM 25752 - ECLIPSE - PIONEER DILUTER-DEMAND OXYGEN REGULATOR WITH SAFETY PRESSURE - TEST OF, 10 April 1946. (Mendelson)

64. X-689 TED NAM 25683 - Oxygen masks, electric heaters for. (Philadelphia)

- Report - TED No. NAM 25683 - HEATER FOR TYPE A-13 OXYGEN MASK, (GENERAL ELECTRIC COMPANY, TYPE P-291-35), 16 November 1945. (Thomas)

- Report - TED No. NAM 25683.1 - TYPE 14 - OXYGEN MASK (GENERAL ELECTRIC COMPANY) TYPE E-1, 16 November 1945. (Thomas)

- Report - TED No. NAM 25683.5 - OXYGEN MASKS, TYPE A-14, TEST OF ELECTRIC HEATER FOR, (GENERAL ELECTRIC COMPANY), 17 May 1946. (Gressly)

65. X-692 TED UNL 25108 - Modification of BuAer M-117 Demand Oxygen mask leak tester. (Pensacola)

- Report No. 1 - MODIFICATION OF BUAER M-117 DEMAND OXYGEN MASK LEAK TESTER, 15 May 1946. (Skow and Vaughan)

66. X-694 TED NAM 259009 - Breathing Machine with standard respiratory patterns - development of. (Philadelphia)

- No report. Work continuing.

67. X-708 TED NAM 25714 - Diluter demand regulators. (Philadelphia)

- Report - TED No. NAM 25714 - ECLIPSE-PIONEER DILUTER DEMAND REGULATORS MODEL 2851-A10 AND 2858-A1 - TEST OF, 11 January 1945. (Harlow and Watts)

- Report - TED No. NAM 25714.1 - DEFECTIVE ECLIPSE-PIONEER DILUTER DEMAND REGULATOR - TEST OF, 22 October 1945. (Perkinson, Jr.)

- Report - (Final) - TED NAM 25714.2 - DEFECTIVE ECLIPSE PIONEER DILUTER DEMAND OXYGEN REGULATORS, FLOWMETER TEST OF, 27 March 1946. (Scott)

68. TED NAM 25268 - Positive Pressure Demand Oxygen Regulator Manufactured by Linde Air Products Co., - Test of. (Philadelphia)

- Report - Same title as above, 17 June 1944. (Watts and Hays)

69. TED NAM 25283 - NDRC Oximeters - NDRC Model 3, Oxygen Want Indicator with Relay and NDRC Flight Research Oximeter Model 14. (Philadelphia)

- Report - TED No. NAM 25283 - N.D.R.C. OXIMETER, 30 March 1944. (Gressly and Meakin)

- Report - TED No. NAM 25283 - N.D.R.C. FLIGHT RESEARCH OXIMETER (MODEL 14, SERIAL NO. 202), 29 August 1944. (Thomas and Ward)

- Report - TED No. NAM 25283 (2) N.D.R.C. OXIMETER - N.D.R.C. MODEL 3, OXYGEN WANT INDICATOR WITH RELAY, 24 August 1944. (Watts)

70. TED NAM 25331 - Oxygen Recharging Trailers. (Philadelphia)

- Report - TED No. NAM 25331.1 - OXYGEN RECHARGING TRAILER MANUFACTURED BY NATIONAL AUTOMATIC TOOL COMPANY, INC., RICHMOND, INDIANA - TEST AND DEVELOPMENT OF, 11 August 1945. (Cherry)

- Report - TED No. NAM 25331.2 - OXYGEN RECHARGING TRAILER ASSEMBLY EMPLOYING MARK III BOMB TRUCK - TEST OF, 11 August 1945. (Cherry)

71. TED NAM 25341 - General Electric Pressure Breathing Oxygen Regulator - Test of. (Philadelphia)

- Report - TED No. NAM 25341 - GENERAL ELECTRIC PRESSURE BREATHING OXYGEN REGULATOR, 24 July 1944. (Watts and Hays)

72. TED NAM 25352 - Helmets, Flying - Oxygen Mask Attachment for - Development of. (Philadelphia)

- Report - TED No. NAM 25352 - Same title as above, 12 August 1944. (Watts and Meakin)

73. TED NAM 25468 - Recording Instrument to Measure Flow and Flow Resistance of Air-Oxygen Mixtures - Development and Test of Laboratory Model. (Philadelphia)

- Report - Same title as above - 12 December 1944. (Watts and Cherry)

- Report - TED No. NAM 25468.1 - PART I - RECORDING INSTRUMENT TO MEASURE FLOW AND FLOW RESISTANCE OF AIR-OXYGEN MIXTURES - DEVELOPMENT AND TEST OF FLIGHT MODEL, 25 April 1946. (Brown)

74. TED NAM 25507 - Aircraft Oxygen Cylinder Valves. (Philadelphia)

- Report - TED No. NAM 25507.1 - REPORT ON AIRCRAFT OXYGEN CYLINDER VALVES - USE OF GRAFOLUX - TEST OF, 14 June 1945. (Hays)

- Report - TED NAM 25507.2 - AIRCRAFT OXYGEN CYLINDER VALVES - LUBRICANTS FOR - TEST OF, 25 January 1946. (Cherry)

75. TED NAM 25551 - Helmets, Flying - Improved Design of - Development and Test of. (Philadelphia)

- Report - TED No. NAM 25551 - Same title as above, 8 February 1946. (Watts)

- Final Report - TED No. NAM 25551 - Same title as above, 22 April 1946. (Scott)

76. TED NAM 25574 - Oxygen Systems for Transport Aircraft - Development of. (Philadelphia)

- Report - Same title as above, 15 February 1946. (Meakin)

77. TED NAM 25646 - Diluter Demand Oxygen Regulator Diaphragm Shield - Evaluation of. (Philadelphia)

- Report - Same title as above, 9 March 1945. (Watts)

78. TED NAM 259002 - Positive Locking Connector for Oxygen Masks - Test of. (Philadelphia)

- Report - TED No. NAM 259002.1 - POSITIVE LOCKING CONNECTOR FOR TYPE A-14 OXYGEN MASK - TEST OF, (JOHNSON FOUNDATION), 20 February 1946. (Meakin)

79. TED NIH 2508 - Tests of the Canadian C3B Air-Oxygen Demand Valve, (NIH)

- Report - Same title as above, 25 February 1946. (Bowen)

80. TED NIH 2510 - Report on Performance of Pioneer Diluter Demand Safety Pressure Regulators. (NIH)

81. TED NIH 2516 - Adaptation of A-14 Mask as a Possible Means of Applying Artificial Respiration.

82. TED NIH 2518 - Individual Oxygen Breathing Devices. (NIH)

- Report, Part I - Same title as above, 10 July 1945. (Bowen, Brubach, and Specht)

- Report, Part II - Same title and authors as above, 10 September 1945.

83. TED PTR 2546 - Trial Aircraft Installation of Individual Diluter Demand Oxygen Units. (Patuxent River)

- Final Report - Same title as above, 15 March 1945. (Eckman and Early)

84. TED PTR 2547 - Oxygen Equipment - Tests of. (Patuxent River)

- Report - (Final) - TED No. PTR 2547 (1) - TEST OF OXYGEN TRANSFER EQUIPMENT - CURTIS COMPRESSOR (CONTRACT Noa(s) 1501) 3 April 1945. (Mathis and Early)

- Report - TED No. PTR 2547 (2) - TESTS OF THE MSA OXYGEN TRANSFER EQUIPMENT, (FINAL REPORT ON), January 1944. (Author unknown)

- Report - (Final) - TED No. PTR 2547 (3) - WIDE-RANGE OXYGEN COMPRESSOR, WALTER KIDDE AND COMPANY, 20 February 1945. (Mathis and Early)

- Report - (Preliminary) - TED No. PTR 2547 (4) - TESTS OF THE LINDE OXYGEN TRANSFER EQUIPMENT, January 1945. (Author unknown)

- Report - (Final) - TED No. PTR 2547 (8) - TESTS OF THE MSA OXYGEN TRANSFER EQUIPMENT TYPE II, 25 April 1945.

85. TED PTR 2593 - Tests of the F4U-ID and F4U-4 Airplanes, Effect of slipstream on Diluter Demand Oxygen Regulator Diaphragm. (Patuxent River)

- Report - TED No. PTR 2593.1 - TESTS OF THE EFFECT OF SLIPSTREAM ON THE DIAPHRAGM OF THE PIONEER DILUTER DEMAND OXYGEN REGULATOR IN THE SB2C-3 AND

- THE TBM-3, 6 June 1945.

86. TED UNL 25165 - Test of Japanese Aviation Oxygen Equipment, (CEE 20349). (Pensacola)

- Report No. 1 - Same title as above, 21 April 1944. (Fugitt)

87. TED UNL 25191 - Army Emergency Breathing Apparatus. T-1 Manufactured by Mine Safety Appliances Company, Test of. (NMRI)

- Memo Report - COMMENT ON THE USE OF THE ARMY EMER GENCY BREATHING APPARATUS T-1 FOR UNDERWATER RESCUE, 22 May 1945. (White, Jr. and Hayter)

88. NMRI-44 - Physiological criteria for the engineering and development of bail-out oxygen equipment. (NMRI)

- Report - Same title as above, 21 February 1944. (Shelesnyak)

- Report - ERRATA IN ABOVE REPORT, 18 July 1944. (No author given)

89. NMRI-55 - Emergency use of the diluter demand oxygen regulator, (Pioneer) by two men. (NMRI)

- Report - Same title as above, 16 March 1944. (King and Shelesnyak)

90. NMRI-61 - Evaluation of methods for cleaning and sterilizing oxygen masks. (NMRI)

- Report - Same title as above, 26 April 1944. (Duggan)

91. NMRI-75 - Evaluation of baralyme as a carbon dioxide absorbent. (NMRI)

- Report - Same title as above, 14 July 1944. (Henson and Pender)

92. NMRI-79 - Simulated high altitude bail-out parachute descent using special breathing procedures and without the use of bail-out oxygen equipment. (NMRI)

- Report - Same title as above, 7 August 1944. (Shelesnyak)

93. NMRI-136 - Cylinder oxygen expenditures of A-12 Diluter Demand Regulators. (NMRI)

- Report - Same title as above, 18 July 1945. (Goldman, King, and Henson)

94. NMRI-149 - Report on a spray method for sterilizing oxygen masks. (NMRI)

- Report - Same title as above, 29 November 1945. (Gillmore and Comploier)

95. Pensacola - Tests on mechanical breathing apparatus. (Pensacola)

- Report No. 1 - (Final) - Same title as above, 1 July 1944. (Gemmill)

96. Pensacola - Testing of Pauling Oxygen Meter, Model P, Serial No. 40. (Pensacola)

- Memorandum Report - Same title as above, 27 November 1944. (Fugitt)

97. Pensacola - Testing of Small Size Pauling Oxygen Meter, Serial A-103. (Pensacola)

- Memorandum Report - Same title as above, 4 January 1945. (No author given)

98. Pensacola - The Use of a Gasoline Rotameter Standard in PBY Aircraft as an Instrument for Metering Oxygen Gas. (Pensacola)

- Report - Same title as above, 20 April 1945. (White)

99. Philadelphia - Continuous Positive Pressure Demand Oxygen Breathing Equipment. (Philadelphia)

- Report - Same title as above, September 1944. (Gressly)

OXYGEN

Leak Testing of Oxygen Masks

1. X-288 - Comparison of Oxygen Mask Leak Testing Methods. (Pensacola)

   - Report No. 1 - (Final) - Subject same as above, 2 April 1944. (Gemmill)

   - Report No. 2 - Subject same as above, 1 July 1944. (Lilienthal, Riley, and Fugitt)

2. X-312 - Evaluation of the McKesson Leak Testing Methods for Oxygen Masks. (NMRI)

   - Report No. 1 - EVALUATION OF THE McKESSON LEAK TESTING METHOD FOR OXYGEN MASKS, 12 April 1944. (Henson, King, and Goldman)

   - Report No. 2 - EVALUATION OF LEAK TESTING METHODS FOR OXYGEN MASKS, 20 June 1944. (Henson, King, and Goldman)

   - Memorandum Report - SIGNIFICANCE OF THE RESULTS OF TESTS FOR OXYGEN MASK LEAKAGE, 4 October 1944. (King)

   - Report X-312A - CALIBRATION OF TWO PLASTIC POCKET LEAK TESTERS, 29 November 1944. (Vollmer and Goldman)

   - Report X-312B - CALIBRATION OF ONE PLASTIC POCKET LEAK TESTER, 15 December 1944. (Vollmer)

   - Report X-312C - CALIBRATION OF TWO McKESSON POCKET MODEL LEAK TESTERS, 16 December 1944. (Vollmer)

3. X-389 - Comparison of Oxygen Mask Leak Testing Without Special Apparatus and by the Scholander Nitrogen Analyzer. (Pensacola)

   - Report No. 1 - Title same as above, 28 May 1944. (Riley and Fugitt)

4. X-422 TED UNL 25108 - Evaluation of Pocket Size Oxygen Mask Leak Tester Manufactured by McKesson Appliances Company. (Pensacola)

- Report No. 1 - (Final) - EVALUATION OF POCKET SIZE OXYGEN MASK LEAK TESTER MANUFACTURED BY McKESSON APPLIANCE COMPANY, 21 August 1944. (Fugitt)

5. X-449 - Evaluation of Pocket Mask Leak Tester, (Leak Tester, demand oxygen Mask, BuAer, M-117) made by Master Plastics Molding Corp. (Pensacola)

- Report No. 1 - Title same as above, 3 August 1944. (Fugitt)

6. X-477 - Evaluation of the Plastic Leak Tester in Comparison with other Methods for Testing Oxygen Mask Leakage. (San Diego)

- Report No. 1 - (Final) - Same title as above. Undated. (Mueller, Pope, Sharpe, Sweeney, Barrington, Yarbrough, Baur, and Ballentine)

7. X-521 - Determination of Negative Pressure in Masks Necessary to Obliterate Leaks. (Pensacola)

- Report No. 1 - A STUDY OF THE MANNER IN WHICH MASK LEAKS CHANGE WITH VARYING NEGATIVE PRESSURES, 29 January 1945. (Fugitt)

8. X-565 - The Constancy of Leakage into Poorly Fitting Masks as Measured with the McKesson Spirometer Type Tester. (Pensacola)

- Report No. 1 - Title same as above, 5 May 1945. (Fugitt)

9. X-665 TED PEN 2504 - RCAF Oxygen Mask Leak Tester, Evaluation of. (Pensacola)

- Report No. 1 - Title same as above, 7 September 1945. (Weatherby)

10. X-698 TED UNL 25108 - Evaluation of Modified Pocket Type Oxygen Mask Leak Tester (McKesson Appliance Company). (Pensacola)

- Report No. 1 - Title same as above, 27 March 1945. (Skow and Vaughan)

11. NMRI-46 - Aperture Method of Stating Oxygen Mask Leakage. (NMRI)

		- Report - Title same as above, 23 February 1944. (King)
12.	Alameda	- Leak Tester to Determine Oxygen Mask Leakage. (Alameda)
		- Memorandum Report - entitled as above, (Scholander and McKesson Testers), 26 February 1944. (Iverson)
13.	Pensacola	- Comparison of Reproducibility of Mask Leak Measurements by the McKesson Method and the Scholander Method. (Pensacola)
		- Memorandum Report - Title same as above, 14 July 1945. (Fugitt and Burt)

OXYGEN

Liquid and Chemical Oxygen

1. X-586 TED UNL 25198 - Evaluation of Chemicals as sources of Oxygen Supply for Aircraft Use. (NMRI)

   - Report No. 1 - CHEMICAL EVALUATION OF THE NAVAL RESEARCH LABORATORY CHLORATE CANDLE, 20 November 1945. (Catchpole and Rohrback - work is continuing)

2. X-618 TED PTR 2547 - Oxygen Equipment, Tests of. (Patuxent River)

   - Report (Final) - TED No. PTR 2547(1) - TEST OF OXYGEN TRANSFER EQUIPMENT - CURTIS COMPRESSOR (CONTRACT NOa(s) 1501)), 3 April 1945. (Mathis and Early)

   - Report - TED No. PTR 2547(2) - TESTS OF THE MSA OXYGEN TRANSFER EQUIPMENT, January 1944, (FINAL REPORT ON). (Author unknown)

   - Report (Final) - TED No. PTR 2547(3) - WIDE-RANGE OXYGEN COMPRESSOR, WALTER KIDDE AND COMPANY, 20 February 1945. (Mathis and Early)

   - Report (Preliminary) - TED No. PTR 2547(4) - TESTS OF THE LINDE OXYGEN TRANSFER EQUIPMENT, January 1945. (Author unknown)

   - Report - TED No. PTR 2457(5) - TESTS OF A. D. LITTLE AND CO. HAND OPERATED LIQUID OXYGEN PUMP, 30 July 1945. (Mathis and Early)

   - Report - TED No. PTR 2547(7) - TESTS OF THE KIDDE OXYGEN TRANSFER EQUIPMENT, 22 June 1945. (Mathis and Early)

   - Report - TED No. PTR 2547.8 - TESTS OF THE MSA OXYGEN TRANSFER EQUIPMENT TYPE II, April 1945. (Author unknown)

   - Report - TED No. PTR 2547.10 and 2547.11 TEST AND EVALUATION OF OXYGEN RECHARGING TRAILERS, 26 October 1945. (Durm and Mathis)

3. X-644 TED UNL 2599 - Liquid Oxygen Aircraft Converters. (Pensacola)

- Report No. 1 - TED No. UNL 2599.1 - LIQUID OXYGEN AIRCRAFT CONVERTERS, AKERMAN 50 LITER UNIT - TEST OF, (PEAK FLOW CHARACTERISTICS), 17 July 1945. (White)

- Report No. 2 - TED No. UNL 2599.1 - LIQUID OXYGEN AIRCRAFT CONVERTERS, AKERMAN FIFTY LITER UNIT - TEST OF (EVAPORATION RATES AND FAILURE OF THE DEWAR CONTAINER), 25 July 1945. (White)

- Report No. 3 - TED No. UNL 2599.1 - SAFETY DEVICE FOR LIQUID OXYGEN CONVERTERS, 20 February 1946. (Weatherby)

- Report No. 1 - TED No. UNL 2599.2 - LIQUID OXYGEN AIRCRAFT CONVERTERS MATHIS-MILAN ITEM II CONTRACT NXs 6139 - TEST OF, 10 October 1944. (White)

4. TED PTR 2522 - Improved Design of Liquid Oxygen Converters. (Mathis-Milan, Patuxent River)

- Report in letter form - Title same as above, 1 March 1944. (Osborne)

5. TED PTR 2567 - Flight tests of Liquid Oxygen Aircraft Converters. (Patuxent River)

- Report (Preliminary) - Same title as above, 28 February 1945. (Mathis and Early)

- Report (Interim) - Same title as above, 10 October 1945.

OXYGEN

Low Pressure Chamber Indoctrination and Training

1. X-38 - Repeat Reliability of Classification Runs in Chamber at 35,000 Feet. (Pensacola)

   - Report - CHANGE IN RESISTANCE TO DECOMPRESSION, November 1942. (No author given - findings published in CAM Report No. 65 dated 18 August 1942.)

   - Final Report - RESEARCH PROJECT REGARDING CLASSIFICATION TESTS IN LOW PRESSURE CHAMBER, undated. (No author given - findings reported in CAM Report No. 89 dated 30 October 1942.)

2. X-501 - Evaluation of Oxygen and Altitude Indoctrination Program. (Norfolk)

   - Report No. 1 - Same title as above. Subtitle: STUDY OF THE ABILITY OF AVIATION PERSONNEL TO LOCATE DEFECTIVE PARTS OF OXYGEN EQUIPMENT, (THE A-12 PIONEER DILUTER DEMAND REGULATOR AND THE A-14 OXYGEN MASK), 7 November 1945. (Dury, Garrett, Carroll and Tabor, Jr.)

   - Report No. 2 - Same title as above. Subtitle: A STUDY OF THE FACTUAL KNOWLEDGE POSSESSED BY AVIATION PERSONNEL CONCERNING THE USE OF OXYGEN AND OXYGEN EQUIPMENT, 7 November 1945. (Carroll, Garrett, Dury, and Tabor, Jr.)

   - Report No. 3 - Same title as above. Subtitle: STUDY OF A PROPOSED PRE-FLIGHT CHECK LIST FOR OXYGEN EQUIPMENT, 7 November 1945. (Dury, Carroll, Garrett, and Tabor, Jr.)

OXYGEN

Physiology

1. X-116 - Pressure breathing (a) Physiology of, and (b) the Testing and Development of Equipment. (NMRI)

- Report No. 1 - PRESSURE BREATHING; Part A. - The Pneumolator. (Ivy) - Part B. - 1. Modified F. W. B. Recirculator. 2. Cyclic Pulmonary Inflation (Experimental), 17 February 1943. (Behnke and Consolazio)

- Report No. 2 - PRESSURE BREATHING OF AIR AT SIMULATED HIGH ALTITUDE, 14 June 1943. (Behnke, White, Pace and Consolazio)

2. X-250 - Studies of Electrolyte Balance of the Body and of Urinary Metabolites Associated with High Altitude and Pilot Fatigue. (NMRI)

- Report No. 1 - THE EFFECT ON THE UREA CLEARANCE OF NORMAL MEN OF ONE HOUR EXPOSURE TO SIMULATED ALTITUDES UP TO 18,000 FEET, 27 October 1945. (Farr, Goldman, Vollmer, Whaley and Henson)

3. X-313 - A study of blood cell volume in relation to the acute physiologic responses to lowered oxygen tensions and the classification of individuals with respect to their tolerance for anoxia. (NMRI)

- Report No. 1 - THE EFFECT OF ACUTE HYPOXIA, WITH AND WITHOUT ADDED CARBON DIOXIDE, ON THE BLOOD CELLS IN MAN, 28 August 1945. (Smith and Pace)

4. X-323 - Correlation of arterial oxygen saturation with concentration of oxygen in inspired air. (Pensacola)

- Report (Preliminary) - THE DETERMINATION OF ARTERIAL OXYGEN SATURATIONS FROM SAMPLES OF "CAPILLARY" BLOOD, 9 February 1944. (Lilienthal and Riley)

- Report No. 2 - THE ACCURACY OF THE SCHOLANDER NITROGEN METHOD IN THE ANALYSIS OF HIGH OXYGEN - LOW NITROGEN GAS MIXTURES AT SEA LEVEL AND AT ALTITUDE, 15 April 1944. (Lilienthal, Riley and Fugitt)

- Report No. 3 - THE DETERMINATION OF ARTERIAL CARBON DIOXIDE CONTENT FROM SAMPLES OF "CAPILLARY" BLOOD, 30 September 1944. (Lilienthal and Riley)

- Report No. 4 - ARTERIAL OXYHEMOGLOBIN SATURATIONS AT CRITICAL PRESSURE-ALTITUDES BREATHING VARIOUS MIXTURES OF OXYGEN AND NITROGEN (WITH A NOTE ON THE EFFECT OF EXERCISE), 12 October 1944. (Riley and Lilienthal)

5. X-373 - Determination of arterial oxygen saturation from samples of capillary blood. (NMRI)

- Report - APPRAISAL OF THE METHOD OF DETERMINING ARTERIAL OXYGEN SATURATION BY USING ARTERIALIZED EAR BLOOD, 13 December 1944. (Pecora and Consolazio)

6. X-396 - Effect of temperature on anoxic failure in naval personnel in altitude chamber. (Miami)

- Report No. 1 - Same title as above, 27 June 1944. (Houston, Cohen, Nuzie and Besson)

- Report No. 2 - Same title as above, 8 August 1944. (Houston, Nuzie, Seitz and Besson)

7. X-402 - Individual variation in respiratory response to carbon dioxide at altitude. (Pensacola)

- Report No. 1 - Same title as above, 25 July 1944. (Weatherby and Burt)

8. X-450 - Development of a simple method for determination of oxygen tension in blood. (Pensacola)

- Report No. 1 - A DIRECT METHOD FOR DETERMINATION OF OXYGEN AND CARBON DIOXIDE TENSIONS IN BLOOD, 9 January 1945. (Riley)

- Report No. 2 - A DIRECT METHOD FOR DETERMINATION OF OXYGEN AND CARBON DIOXIDE TENSIONS IN BLOOD, 16 July 1945. (Riley)

9. X-475 - Determination of aqueous vapor tension in expired air. (Pensacola)

- No report - work continuing.

10. X-484 - The physiological effects of anoxia and exercise. (Pensacola)

- Report No. 1 - THE PHYSIOLOGICAL EFFECTS OF ANOXIA AND EXERCISE. Subtitle: THE RELATIONSHIP BETWEEN ALVEOLAR AIR OXYGEN TENSIONS AND ARTERIAL BLOOD OXYGEN SATURATIONS, 15 May 1945. (Gemmill and Malone)

- Report No. 2 - ON THE DETERMINATION OF THE PHYSIOLOGICALLY EFFECTIVE PRESSURES OF OXYGEN AND CARBON DIOXIDE IN ALVEOLAR AIR, 22 January 1946. (Riley and Lilienthal)

- Report No. 3 - AN EXPERIMENTAL ANALYSIS IN MAN OF THE OXYGEN PRESSURE GRADIENT FROM ALVEOLAR AIR TO ARTERIAL BLOOD DURING REST AND EXERCISE AT SEA LEVEL AND AT ALTITUDE, 23 February 1946. (Lilienthal and Riley)

- Work is continuing.

11. X-490 - A study of oxygen and carbon dioxide dissociation curves in vivo under normal conditions and during anoxia and acapnia, with simultaneous studies of neuro-muscular excitability. (Pensacola)

- Report No. 1 - THE RELATIONSHIPS OF OXYGEN, CARBON DIOXIDE AND HEMOGLOBIN IN THE BLOOD OF MAN: OXYHEMOGLOBIN DISSOCIATION UNDER VARIOUS PHYSIOLOGICAL CONDITIONS, 11 September 1945. (Riley and Lilienthal)

12. X-500 TED UNL 25113 - Evaluation of complete inspiratory obstruction as a warning of failure of oxygen supply to a demand regulator. (Pensacola)

- Report No. 1 - APPRAISAL OF COMPLETE INSPIRATORY OBSTRUCTION AS A WARNING OF OXYGEN SUPPLY FAILURE: COMPARISON OF THE A12 AND THE CANADIAN C-3B REGULATOR, 13 January 1945. (Weatherby and Burt)

13. X-524 - Transfusion of human erythrocytes as a possible means of increasing tolerance to hypoxia. (NMRI)

- Report No. 1 - PRELIMINARY STUDIES ON THE TRANSFUSION OF RED BLOOD CELLS INTO NORMAL MEN IN ORDER TO INCREASE TOLERANCE TO HYPOXIA, 9 March 1945. (Pace, Consolazio and Lozner)

- Work is continuing.

14. X-572 - The rates of fall of blood oxygen saturation at simulated altitudes following mask removals. (Pensacola)

- Report No. 1 (Preliminary) - THE RATES OF FALL OF BLOOD OXYGEN SATURATIONS AT SIMULATED ALTITUDES FOLLOWING MASK REMOVALS (PERIOD OF USEFUL CONSCIOUSNESS FOLLOWING MASK REMOVALS AT A SIMULATED ALTITUDE OF THIRTY THOUSAND FEET), 26 July 1945. (White)

- Report No. 1 - THE RATES OF FALL OF BLOOD OXYGEN SATURATION AT SIMULATED ALTITUDES FOLLOWING MASK REMOVALS. Subtitle: PERIOD OF USEFUL CONSCIOUSNESS AND TIME TO IMMINENT UNCONSCIOUSNESS FOLLOWING CHANGE FROM 100% OXYGEN TO AMBIENT AIR AT ALTITUDES ABOVE 28,000 FEET, 1 December 1945. (Hoffman, Clark, Jr., and Brown, Jr.)

15. X-579 - Investigation of isothermal expansion of gases saturated with water vapor. (Pensacola)

- Report No. 1 - ISOTHERMAL EXPANSION OF GASES SATURATED WITH WATER VAPOR, 2 May 1945. (Fugitt)

16. X-616 TED UNL 25113 - Reaction of aviation personnel at simulated altitude to inspiratory obstruction. (Norfolk)

- Report - REACTION OF AVIATION PERSONNEL AT A SIMULATED ALTITUDE OF 30,000 FEET TO INSPIRATORY OBSTRUCTION, 16 November 1945. (Dury, Garrett and Tabor)

17. X-675 - Relation of pulmonary ventilation to arterial oxygen saturation. (Pensacola)

- Report No. 1 - Same title as above, 15 December 1945. (Houston and Nez)

- Report No. 2 - RELATION OF PULMONARY VENTILATION TO ARTERIAL OXYGEN TENSION, 20 January 1946. (Houston and Nez)

- Work is continuing.

18. X-714 - Studies in respiration and the physiological requirements for oxygen equipment. (NMRI)

- No report - work is continuing.

19. NMRI-51 - Development of a burette for analyzing high concentrations of oxygen in gas mixtures. (NMRI)

- Report - Same title as above, 27 April 1944. (Consolazio and Pecora)

20. Pensacola - The effect of decreased barometric pressure, anoxia, cold and protective devices upon navigating efficiency. (Pensacola)

- Report - Same title as above, May 1943. (No author given)

Voluntary Pressure Breathing and Hyperventilation

21. X-198 - Pressure breathing of ambient air at altitudes without aid of a special device. (Pensacola and Corpus Christi)

- Pensacola Report No. 1 (Preliminary) - Title same as above, 20 October 1943. (Gemmill, Lilienthal and Riley)

- Pensacola Report No. 2 (Final) - PRESSURE BREATHING WITHOUT THE AID OF A SPECIAL DEVICE: CIRCULATORY MEASUREMENTS AND AN EVALUATION OF THE METHOD FOR SERVICE USE, 10 December 1943. (Lilienthal and Riley)

- Corpus Christi Report - VOLUNTARY PRESSURE BREATHING OF AMBIENT ATMOSPHERE AS A MEANS OF INCREASING THE OXYGEN SATURATION OF THE BLOOD, 19 October 1943. (Commoner)

- Corpus Christi Report - A TRAINING MANUAL FOR THE EMERGENCY BREATHING PROCEDURE, 19 May 1944. (Commoner)

- Corpus Christi Report - FLIGHT TESTS OF THE EMERGENCY BREATHING PROCEDURE, 22 June 1944. (Commoner)

- Corpus Christi Report - THE VALUE OF HYPERVENTILATION AS A MEANS OF SURVIVING HIGH-ALTITUDE EMERGENCIES WITHOUT OXYGEN: A COMPARISON WITH THE EMERGENCY BREATHING PROCEDURE, 31 July 1944. (Commoner)

22. X-291 - Voluntary pressure breathing, physiological appraisal of. (NMRI)

- Report No. 1 - EVALUATION OF THE EMERGENCY BREATHING PROCEDURE (VOLUNTARY PRESSURE BREATHING), 30 June 1944. (King, Goldman, Henson and Whaley)

23. X-343 - Physiological evaluation of voluntary pressure breathing. (Miami)

- Report No. 1 - EVALUATION OF EMERGENCY BREATHING PROCEDURE AT 25,000 FEET, 8 July 1944. (Houston, Nuzie, Seitz and Besson)

- Report No. 2 - EVALUATION OF HYPERVENTILATION OF AMBIENT AIR AT 25,000 FEET, 25 August 1944. (Houston, Nuzie, Seitz, Besson and Young)

- Report No. 3 - COMPARISON OF VOLUNTARY PRESSURE BREATHING AND MODIFIED HYPERVENTILATION AT 25,000 FEET IN THE CHAMBER AND IN OPERATIONAL AIRCRAFT, 8 September 1944. (Houston, Nuzie, Seitz, Besson and Young)

- Report No. 4 - EVALUATION OF THE EMERGENCY BREATHING PROCEDURE. Subtitle: CONTROL STUDY: DURATION OF CONSCIOUSNESS AT ALTITUDES BETWEEN 19,000 and 22,000 FEET, 5 January 1946. (Houston)

24. X-454 - Hyperventilation breathing air as a means of maintaining consciousness at 25,000 feet. (Pensacola)

- Report No. 1 (Final) - Title same as above, 30 September 1944. (Riley, Lilienthal and Fugitt)

OXYGEN

Positive Pressure Breathing Equipment

1. X-303 - Altitude pressure bag, physiological evaluation of. (NMRI)

   - Report - Title same as above, 22 March 1944. (King and Futcher)

2. X-631 TED NAM 25362 - Positive pressure breathing equipment. (Philadelphia)

   - Report - TED No. NAM 25362 - POSITIVE PRESSURE BREATHING EQUIPMENT, DEVELOPMENT AND TEST OF, 4 September 1944. (Gressly)

   - Report - TED No. NAM 25362.1 - POSITIVE PRESSURE BREATHING EQUIPMENT - INDOCTRINATION AND TRAINING IN USE OF, 29 October 1945. (Scott)

   - Report - TED No. NAM 25362.2 - OXYGEN PRESSURE REDUCER (SERIAL No. YS-69-1) AND 30.5 CUBIC INCH HIGH PRESSURE OXYGEN BOTTLE (SERIAL No. K77914S) FOR BAIL-OUT SYSTEMS MANUFACTURED BY LINDE AIR PRODUCTS COMPANY - TESTS OF, 10 October 1944. (Hays and Watts)

   - Report - TED No. NAM 25362.3 - Y CONNECTOR WITH INTERLOCKING CHECK VALVES SERIAL No. YS-65-2, DM587 BY LINDE AIR PRODUCTS CO. - TESTS OF, 10 October 1944. (Hays and Watts)

   - Report - TED No. NAM 25362.4 - POSITIVE PRESSURE BREATHING EQUIPMENT - DEVELOPMENT AND TEST OF PHASE 4 - PRESSURE VEST TEST, 3 August 1945. (Mendelson)

   - Report - TED No. NAM 25362.6 - OXYGEN PRESSURE BREATHING EQUIPMENT - FLIGHT TEST OF, 27 November 1945. (Scott)

   - Report - TED No. NAM 25362.7 - POSITIVE PRESSURE BREATHING EQUIPMENT - INDIVIDUAL KIT - DEVELOPMENT OF, 15 June 1945. (Meakin)

   - Report - TED No. NAM 25362.8 - POSITIVE PRESSURE BREATHING EQUIPMENT - QUICK DISCONNECT COUPLING - TEST OF, 27 June 1945. (Meakin)

- Report - TED No. NAM 25362.9 - PRESSURE BREATHING OXYGEN MASKS, A. M. L. LEAK TESTER, 31 July 1945. (Meakin)

- Report - TED No. NAM 25362.10 - POSITIVE PRESSURE OXYGEN BREATHING EQUIPMENT - SPRING LOADED INHALATION VALVES - DEVELOPMENT AND TEST OF, 11 October 1945. (Perkinson, Jr.)

3. NAES

- Continuous positive pressure demand oxygen breathing equipment. (Philadelphia)

- Report - Same title as above, September 1944. (Gressly)

J. PHARMACOLOGY

1. X-120 - Field Study of the Effects of benzedrine on small arms firing under conditions of acute fatigue. (Camp Lejeune)

   - Report - FIELD STUDY OF THE EFFECTS OF BENZEDRINE ON SMALL ARMS FIRING UNDER CONDITIONS OF ACUTE FATIGUE, 2 June 1943. (Corey and Webster)

2. X-213 - Effects of scopolamine on marksmanship. (Camp Lejeune)

   - Report - Same title as above. Undated. (Corey and Webster)

K. PHYSICAL FITNESS

1. X-36 - Physical Fitness tests. (Experimental Diving Unit, Navy Yard, Washington, D. C. and NMRI)

- Report - A STEP-UP TEST FOR THE EVALUATION OF CARDIOVASCULAR FUNCTION IN TERMS OF PULSE RATE, AND FOR THE ESTIMATION OF MUSCULAR ENDURANCE, December 1942. (Behnke and Pace)

- Report - ADDITIONAL DATA ON THE STEP-UP TEST TO EVALUATE CARDIOVASCULAR FUNCTION AND MUSCULAR PERFORMANCE. Undated. (Welham, White, Jr. and Behnke)

2. X-709 - Physical Fitness Test, Development of, including Establishment of Standards of Fitness for Naval Personnel. (Pensacola)

- No report. Work continuing.

L. SAFETY DEVICES AND SURVIVAL HUMAN FACTORS IN ENGINEERING DESIGN

1. X-109
   - Stretcher, Modification of. (NMRI)
   - Report No. 1 - SEMI-RIGID CANVAS LITTERS . . . EXPERIMENTAL STUDY, 5 May 1943. (Mathieson and Duncan)
   - Un-numbered report - COMMENT AND NOTES ON THE TESTING OF SAMPLE LAMINATED WOOD-PLASTIC STRETCHER, 5 September 1944. (Shelesnyak and Margolis)
   - Report - X109A - IMPROVISED STOKES STRETCHER FLOATS FOR AIR/SEA RESCUE, 5 December 1944. (Jennings and Shelesnyak)
   - Report - X109B - EVALUATION OF THE INTERNATIONAL LATEX CORPORATION RAFT FOR STOKES STRETCHER, 5 March 1945. (Jennings)
   - Report - X109C - TESTS ON PLASTIC LITTER DEVELOPED BY SPECIAL DEVICES DIVISION, BUREAU OF AERONAUTICS, 17 May 1945. (Jennings)
   - Report - X109D - A MODIFICATION OF THE SEMI-RIGID CANVAS LITTER (NMRI MODEL A), STOCK No. S6-691, SUPPLY CATALOG, MEDICAL DEPARTMENT, U. S. NAVY, 11 August 1945. (Jennings)
   - Report - X109E - EMPTY AMMUNITION CONTAINERS FOR EMERGENCY FLOTATION, 29 August 1945. (Jennings)
   - Report - X109F - CARRYING STRAPS FOR POLE LITTERS. 7 January 1946. (Jennings)
   - Report - X109G - REPORT ON ORIGINAL MODEL AND MODIFICATION OF THE ELLIS FLOTATION STRETCHER, 1 March 1946. (Jennings)
2. X-115
   - Study of Crash injuries. (Pensacola)
   - This project was transferred to Safety Division, Bureau of Aeronautics.
3. X-292
   - Comparison of different types of parachute harness with particular reference to ease of release. (Pensacola)

- Report No. 1 - Same title as above, 7 March 1944. (Gemmill, Stilwell, Dietz, Riley, Zwierlein, Lawrence, and Fugitt)

4. X-371 - Design of individual (personal) first aid kit for aviation personnel. (NMRI)

- Report - Same title as above, 31 May 1944. (Shelesnyak and Margolis)

5. X-447 - Cardboard Splints, Testing of. (NMRI)

- Report - TESTING OF CARDBOARD SPLINTS, 10 August 1944. (Turner)

6. X-549 - Investigation of pilot seating discomfort. (NMRI and Patuxent)

- Report No. 1 - (TED PTR No. 25124) - INVESTIGATION OF COCKPIT SEATING - EVALUATION OF THE BUAER PILOT SEAT PAN (SP-1) AND BACK PAD (BP-1), THE NIAGARA UNITS GYRATORY SEAT. THE NAVY STANDARD HAIR SEAT AND BACK CUSHION, 6 February 1946. (White, Whitley, and MacGregor)

7. X-554 - Kit, First Aid, camouflaged, for pneumatic life rafts, aeronautic. (NMRI)

- Report No. 1 - DESIGN OF A FIRST AID KIT FOR USE ON PNEUMATIC LIFE RAFTS, 17 April 1945. (Shelesnyak)

- Supplementary Report - TENTATIVE SPECIFICATION, KITS, FIRST AID, CAMOUFLAGED, FOR PNEUMATIC LIFE RAFTS, 17 April 1945. This was prepared in collaboration with the Material Division, Bureau of Medicine and Surgery.

8. X-557 - To prepare medical pouch for air-sea rescue. (Pensacola)

- Report No. 1 - PREPARATION OF A MEDICAL POUCH FOR AIR-SEA RESCUE, 5 May 1945. (Grossman)

9. X-630 - Studies of the biomechanics of aviation crash injuries and of protective measures. (NMRI)

- Report No. 1 - STATIC LOADING TESTS OF LAP SAFETY BELTS AND SHOULDER HARNESSES (NAF-1201-1), 28 August 1945. (Bierman)

- Report No. 2 - Same title as Report No. 1, 27 October 1945. (Bierman)

- Report No. 3 - DESIGN OF AN IMPACT DECELERATOR, 30 November 1945. (Bierman)

- Report No. 4 - DISTRIBUTION OF IMPACT FORCES ON THE HUMAN THROUGH RESTRAINING DEVICES, 21 March 1946. (Bierman and Larsen)

10. X-647 - Altitude, velocity, and time relationships for free falls and parachute descents from aircraft. (Biodynamics Branch, Research Division, BuMed)

- No report. Work continuing.

11. X-651 - Human factors in the design, placement and operation of instruments and controls in aircraft. (NMRI, Patuxent, and Oceana)

- R port No. 1 - MEASUREMENTS OF AIRCREWMEN AND AIRCREW SPACES IN NAVAL AIRCRAFT, 13 December 1945. (King, Vollmer, Henson, Margolis, Pfaffman, Whaley, Newton, and Lewis)

- Report No. 2 - FREEDOM OF MOVEMENT AND PERFORMANCE OF AIRCREWMEN IN RELATION TO AIRCRAFT SPACE AN SIZE OF THE MAN, 19 December 1945. (Vollmer, Henson, Pfaffman, Margolis, King, Selover, Newton, and Kontakevich)

- Memorandum Report - COMMENTS ON AIR SPEED INDICATOR, MANUFACTURER'S PART NO. AW-2 3/4-20-D, U. S. Gauge Company, NP-9-AY, 11 January 1946. (King)

- Memorandum Report - Summary Report to 20 February 1946, 25 February 1946. (Lawrence)

- Memorandum Report - REPORT ON A VISIT TO SPECIAL DEVICES SECTION, ORI, PORT WASHINGTON, N. Y., 13 May 1946. (King)

12. X-660 - Physiological effects of vibration. (NMRI and NRL)

- No report. Work continuing.

13. X-677 - Investigation of safety factors in escape from aircraft. (Cherry Point)

- No report. Work continuing.

14. X-691 - Comparison of flotation characteristics of various types of life preservers. (NMRI)

  - No report. Work continuing.

15. X-695 - Analysis of a random sample of Navy Air-Sea Rescues. (Pensacola)

  - Report No. 1 - Same title as above, January 1946. (Harrison)

16. X-707 - Comparison of flotation characteristics of various types of life preservers. (Sub Base, New London)

  - No report. Work continuing.

17. X-716 - Physiological limits of escape from aircraft. (Biodynamics Branch, Research Division, BuMed)

  - No report. Work continuing.

M. SPEECH INTELLIGIBILITY AND AUDIBILITY

1. X-123 - Improvement of Intercommunication systems. (Pensacola)

   - Report No. 1 - REPORT ON SPEECH INTELLIGIBILITY, 1942. (Steer)

   - Report No. 2 - INTER-COMMUNICATION, IMPROVEMENT OF, INTELLIGIBILITY OF, 28 September 1943. (Steer)

   - Report No. 3 - INTER-COMMUNICATION IMPROVEMENT AND INTELLIGIBILITY OF, 2 October 1943. (Steer)

2. X-322 TED UNL 2575 - Evaluation of gosport speaking tube, contract No. NXsa36914. (Pensacola)

   - Report - (Final) - EVALUATION OF GOSPORT SPEAKING TUBE, 29 July 1944. (Steer and Lawrence)

3. X-520 - Listening training aids for pre-flight and primary flight students. (Pensacola)

   - Report No. 1 - Same title as above, 22 September 1945. (Steer, Hadley, and Kerr)

4. X-634 - Evaluation of Gleason gosport mouthpiece. (Pensacola)

   - Report No. 1 - Same title as above, 18 December 1945. (Steer, Hadley, and Kerr)

5. X-645 - Development and evaluation of techniques to measure speech intelligibility for flight personnel. (Pensacola)

   - Report No. 1 - Same title as above, 5 February 1946. (Steer, Hadley, and Kelly)

6. TED UNL #3111 - Testing of the M-5A/UR lip Microphone. (Pensacola)

   - Report No. 1 - TED UNL No. 3111 - TESTING OF THE M-5A/UR Lip Microphone, January 1945. (Author unknown)

   - Report No. 2 - TED UNL No. 3111 - Same title as Report No. 1, 24 January 1945. (Steer, Hadley, and Kerr)

   - Report No. 3 - TED UNL No. 3111 - Same title as above, 15 February 1945. (Steer, Hadley, and Kerr)

- Report No. 4 - TED UNL No. 3111 - Same title as above, 17 February 1945. (Steer, Hadley, and Kerr)

- Report No. 1 - TED No. UNL 3118 - DETERMINATION OF THE ADAPTABILITY OF M-5A/UR LIP MICROPHONE FOR MOUNTING ON LEFT SIDE EARPHONE SOCKET, 8 March 1946. (Hadley and Kerr)

7. TED UNL 3115 - Acoustical performance of earphone sockets in new helmets; evaluation of in Voice Communication Laboratory. (Pensacola)

- Report No. 1 - EVALUATION OF AVIATION HELMETS - SIZING, 20 August 1945. (Steer, Hadley, Vinacke, and Kerr)

- Report No. 2 - PILOTS' EVALUATION OF AVIATION HELMETS, 28 August 1945. (Steer, Hadley, Vinacke, and Kerr)

- Report No. 3 - ACOUSTICAL PERFORMANCE OF EARPHONE SOCKETS: ATTENUATION AND INSULATION PROPERTIES, 18 October 1945. (Steer, Hadley, and Kerr)

8. TED NAM 3191 - Sonotone Sound Powered Throat Microphone, SP-17-1, Serial No. 60. (Philadelphia)

- Report - Subject title, 26 February 1944. (Newman)

N. TOXIC GASES

1. X-129

- Effects of blood concentrations of carbon monoxide on altitude tolerance. (Pensacola)
- Report No. 1 - (Part I) - THE EFFECT OF VARYING PARTIAL PRESSURE OF OXYGEN AND CARBON MONOXIDE ON THE UPTAKE OF CARBON MONOXIDE IN MAN WITH A NOTE ON THE NBS ANALYZER FOR ALVEOLAR COMPANY, 15 October 1943. (Lilienthal and Pine)
- Addendum to Report No. 1 - Same title as Report No. 1, 11 May 1944. (Same authors)
- Report No. 2 - THE EFFECT OF LOW CONCENTRATIONS OF CARBOXYHEMOGLOBIN UPON THE "ALTITUDE TOLERANCE" OF MAN, 6 March 1944. (Lilienthal and Fugitt)
- Report No. 3 - (Final) - A. THE CONCENTRATION OF CARBON MONOXIDE IN VARIOUS TRAINING AIRCRAFT. B. THE BLOOD CONCENTRATION OF CARBOXY-HEMOGLOBIN IN PERSONNEL IN VARIOUS TRAINING AIRCRAFT, 9 March 1944. (Gemmill, Bierman, Lilienthal, and Fugitt)

2. X-154

- Study of ventilation problems on Hangar Decks of naval carrier vessels. (NMRI)
- The title of this project was changed by official letter dated 15 June 1943, namely: DETERMINATION OF CARBON MONOXIDE AND NOXIOUS GAS CONCENTRATIONS IN AIRCRAFT CARRIER HANGAR DECK SPACE - PLANE WARM-UP.
- Report No. 1 - CO TESTS ABOARD AIRCRAFT CARRIERS, 6 April 1943. (Behnke, Houghton, Consolazio, and Pace) (U. S. S. CARD.)
- Report No. 2 - GAS MASKS AND RESPIRATORS SUITABLE FOR USE IN DIESEL ENGINE FUMES IN THE TANK CARGO SPACE OF LST SHIPS, 5 April 1943. (Houghton, Consolazio, and Pace) This study initiated by the Air Conditioning Sec. of BuShips.
- Report No. 2 - CO TESTS ABOARD AIRCRAFT CARRIERS-USS COWPENS, 15 July 1943. (Behnke, Houghton, White, and Davis)

- Letter report from Air Conditioning Sec. BuShips to Carrier Construction Sec. and Carrier Maintenance Sec., BuShips - Subj: CVE55 Class- CO CONCENTRATIONS AND PSYCHROMETRIC CHANGES IN THE HANGAR SPACE, 3 December 1943. (Houghton)

- Report X-154A - REPORT OF AN INVESTIGATION OF CARBON MONOXIDE CONCENTRATION IN THE HANGAR SPACE AND READY ROOM OF ESCORT AIRCRAFT CARRIER USS NATOMA BAY (CVE-62), 27 December 1943. (Behnke, Houghton, and Pace)

- Report X-154B - REPORT OF AN INVESTIGATION OF CARBON MONOXIDE CONCENTRATION IN THE HANGAR SPACE AND A READY ROOM OF AIRCRAFT CARRIER USS FRANKLIN, (CV-13), 9 May 1944. (Behnke, Houghton, Consolazio, and Pace)

- Report X-154C - REPORT ON THE MEDICAL ASPECTS OF CARBON MONOXIDE CONCENTRATIONS ABOARD THE LST 544 DURING THE WARM-UP OF TANK ENGINES, 7 February 1945. (Behnke, Pace, Consolazio, Pecora, and Pitts)

- Report X-154D - REPORT ON THE MEDICAL ASPECTS OF CARBON MONOXIDE CONCENTRATIONS ABOARD THE AIRCRAFT CARRIER USS BLOCK ISLAND (CVE-106), 11 April 1945. (Behnke, Pace, and Consolazio)

- Report X-154E - AN INVESTIGATION OF CARBON MONOXIDE CONCENTRATION IN THE HANGAR SPACE, READY ROOMS AND OTHER SHIP'S COMPARTMENTS DURING WARM-UP TESTS ON THE AIRCRAFT CARRIER USS MIDWAY (CVB-41), 7 February 1946. (Consolazio, Pecora, and Pitts)

- Work continuing.

3. X-361 - Carbon monoxide determinations in the F4U. (San Diego)

- Report No. 1 - (Final) - Same title as above, Undated. (Mueller, Pope, Jones, Sharpe, Vollmer, and Walker)

4. X-362 - Comparison of MSA Portable Hopcalite Carbon Monoxide Indicator and Bulb Type Colorimeter. (San Diego)

- Report No. 1 - (Final) - Same title as above, March 1944. (Mueller, Pope, Sharpe, Vollmer, and Walker)

5. X-409 - In vivo equilibrium between oxy-, carboxy-, and reduced hemoglobin in blood of human subjects. (Pensacola)

- Report No. 1 - THE RELATIONSHIPS IN VIVO BETWEEN CARBON MONOXIDE, OXYGEN, AND HEMOGLOBIN IN THE BLOOD OF MAN AT ALTITUDE, 20 August 1945. (Lilienthal and Riley)

6. X-417
TED PTR 2568 - Determination of allowable safe limits of carbon monoxide concentrations in aircraft. (NMRI and Patuxent River)

- Report - CO TESTS CONDUCTED AT THE CHANCE-VOUGHT AIRCRAFT PLANT, 18-19 July 1944, 5 August 1944. (Behnke)

- Report No. 1 - THE RATE OF BLOOD ABSORPTION OF LOW CONCENTRATIONS OF CARBON MONOXIDE IN AMBIENT AIR AT SIMULATED ALTITUDES UP TO 10,000 FEET - A SUMMARY OF THE ESSENTIAL DATA, 25 August 1944. (Pace, Consolazio, Pitts, and Pecora)

- Report No. 2 - Same title as No. 1, 31 August 1944. (Pace, Consolazio, Pitts, and Pecora)

- Report No. 3 - THE RELATIONSHIP BETWEEN VARIOUS LEVELS OF COHB IN THE BLOOD AND THE EQUIVALENT PHYSIOLOGICAL ALTITUDE, 30 October 1944. (Pitts and Pace)

- Report No. 4 - A CONTINUOUS SAMPLING DEVICE FOR GASES IN AMBIENT AIR, 15 February 1945. (Goldman and Mathis)

- Supplement to Report No. 4 - METHOD OF REMOVING GAS FOR ANALYSIS FROM COLLECTING CYLINDER OF A CONTINUOUS FLOW SAMPLING DEVICE, 28 March 1945. (Goldman and Consolazio)

- Report No. 5 - THE EVALUATION OF METHODS FOR DETERMINING THE CONCENTRATION OF CARBON MONOXIDE, 23 February 1945. (Consolazio, Pecora, MacDonald, Collison, Kreuger, Platt, O'Neal, and Rae)

- Report No. 6 - THE RATE OF BLOOD ABSORPTION OF LOW CONCENTRATIONS OF CARBON MONOXIDE AT SEA LEVEL, 26 February 1945. (Pitts and Pace)

- Report No. 7 - THE EFFECTS OF CARBON MONOXIDE ON THREE TYPES OF PERFORMANCE AT SIMULATED ALTITUDES OF 10,000 AND 15,500 FEET, 27 February 1945. (Vollmer, King, Fisher, and Birren)

- Report - METHOD OF REMOVING GAS FOR ANALYSIS FROM COLLECTING CYLINDER OF A CONTINUOUS FLOW SAMPLING DEVICE, 28 March 1945. (Goldman and Consolazio)

- Report No. 8 - A NOMOGRAPH FOR THE ESTIMATION OF THE UPTAKE OF CARBON MONOXIDE BY THE BLOOD OF FLYING PERSONNEL, 18 July 1945. (Pace)

- Report No. 9 - A NOMOGRAPH FOR THE ESTIMATION OF THE UPTAKE OF CARBON MONOXIDE BY FLYING PERSONNEL BREATHING AIR OR BREATHING THROUGH A DILUTER DEMAND REGULATOR, 9 August 1945. (Pace)

- Report No. 10 - AN EVALUATION OF THE SJOSTRAND CARBON MONOXIDE INDICATOR, 15 May 1946. (Pecora and Consolazio)

- Memorandum Report - TED PTR 2568 - THE CARBON MONOXIDE CONTENT IN PILOT'S BLOOD RESULTING FROM CARBON MONOXIDE IN THE AIRPLANE COCKPIT DURING FLIGHT, 27 October 1944. (McDonald)

7. X-463 - Toxic gases from assisted take-off units (JATO). (NMRI)

- Report No. 1 - TOXIC GASES FROM ASSISTED TAKE-OFF UNITS, (JATO), 11 October 1944. (Turner, Consolazio, and Gersh)

8. X-555 - AML Blood Carbon Monoxide analyzer, test of. (Pensacola)

- Report No. 1 - TEST OF THE AML BLOOD CARBON MONOXIDE ANALYZER, 25 April 1945. (Lilienthal)

- Report No. 2 - EVALUATION OF THE NIH MIDGET PHOTOMETER FOR THE ESTIMATION OF CARBOXY-HEMOGLOBIN, 29 June 1945. (Lilienthal)

9. X-649 - Carbon monoxide Indicator, MSA Part Number 44170: Test of. (Philadelphia)

- Interim Report - Same title as above, 1 August 1945. (Scott)

- Report - TED No. NAM 25747 - Same title as above, 28 January 1946. (Mendelson)

10. X-657 TED PTR 2594 - MSA HEATED HOPCALITE CO INDICATOR, TEST OF. (Patuxent River)

- Report - (Final) - TED No. PTR 2594 - Same title as above, 10 August 1945. (Mathis)

11. TED NIH 2514 - A simplified photoelectric colorimeter for blood analysis. (NIH)

- Report - Same title as above, 27 September 1944. (Andrews and Horecker)

- Memorandum Report - MIDGET PHOTOMETER FOR BLOOD GAS ANALYSES - COMMENT, 11 October 1944. (Consolazio)

12. TED PTR 2591 - Continuous sampling method of carbon monoxide testing. (Patuxent River)

- Report - TED No. PTR 2591 - Same title as above, 15 April 1946. (Eckman and Commoner)

13. NMRI-69 - Preservation of blood containing carbon monoxide for transportation from the field to the laboratory. (NMRI)

- Report - Same title as above, 6 June 1944. (Consolazio and Pecora)

14. NMRI-90 - EVALUATION OF A MIDGET PHOTOMETER FOR DETERMINING HbCO. (NMRI)

- Report - Same title as above, 22 November 1944. (Consolazio)

15. NMRI-146 - RE-EVALUATION OF THE NIH MIDGET PHOTOMETER FOR DETERMINING CARBOXYHEMOGLOBIN AND TOTAL HEMOGLOBIN. (NMRI)

- Report - Same title as above, 25 September 1945. (Pitts)

16. Pensacola - Test of the NBS method for analysis of carbon monoxide in gas mixtures. (Pensacola)

- Memorandum Report - Same title as above, 26 September 1944. (Fugitt and Lilienthal)

O. VISION

Aircraft and Instrument Lighting

1. X-69 - Comparison of ultra-violet fluorescent maps and maps illuminated with red lights as to discrimination of detail and effect on dark adaptation. (NIH)

   - Preliminary Report - (Letter form) - Subject: THE RELATIVE MERITS OF FLUORESCENT AND RED LIGHTING OF AERONAUTICAL CHARTS, 14 September 1942. (Lee and Weinbach)

   - Letter Report - Subject: LIGHT ADAPTATION THROUGH EXPOSURE FOR VARIOUS LENGTHS OF TIME TO A RED GLARE SOURCE, 11 December 1942. (Lee)

   - Letter Report - Subject: LIGHTING OF AERONAUTICAL CHARTS. COMPARISON OF THE EFFECT ON DARK ADAPTATION OF EXPOSURES OF VARYING DURATIONS TO RED AND WHITE GLARE SOURCES OF THE SAME BRIGHTNESS, 23 January 1943. (Lee)

2. X-498 - Investigation of visual factors contributing to night aircraft accidents, with special reference to methods of lighting planes. (Corpus Christi)

   - Report No. 1 - Same title as above, 16 July 1945. (Walker)

   - Report No. 2 - Same title as above, 15 October 1945. (Walker)

3. X-562 - An analysis of night accidents in relation to the illumination afforded by varying degrees of moonlight. (Pensacola)

   - Report No. 1 - AN ANALYSIS OF NIGHT ACCIDENTS IN RELATION TO CHANGES IN ILLUMINATION RESULTING FROM THE LUNAR CYCLE, 6 August 1945. (Pfaffman, Fosberg, and Bugelski)

4. X-636 - A comparison of ultra-violet and indirect red systems of illumination for airplane instrument panels. (Philadelphia)

   - Report - TED No. NAM 4422 - Same title as above, 11 July 1945. (Bromer)

VISION - COLOR VISION

1. X-42
   - Trial of Canadian Navy colour vision lantern in comparison with other tests of color vision. (N.L.)
   - Report - (Preliminary) - COLOR VISION TESTING, 12 September 1942. (Shilling)
   - Report - TRIAL OF ROYAL CANADIAN NAVY COLOUR VISION LANTERN IN COMPARISON WITH OTHER TESTS OF COLOR VISION, 18 January 1943. (Shilling)

2. X-75
   - Color perception test, preliminary design of. (Pensacola)
   - Report - Same title as above, 15 February 1943. (No author given)

3. X-225
   - Test of the Williams Lantern for color perception. (New London)
   - Report - COLOR VISION REPORT No. 6, 22 November 1943. (Author unknown)

4. X-261
   - Study of the effects of certain illuminants on scores made on Pseudo-isochromatic tests. (New London)
   - Report - COLOR VISION REPORT No. 4, 22 November 1943. (Farnsworth)

5. X-262
   - Analysis of construction of Pseudo-isochromatic plates with reference to illumination. (New London)
   - Report - COLOR VISION REPORT No. 5, January 1944. (Farnsworth)

6. X-263
   - The critical hue regions of transmission of illuminant A for Deuteranamalous and Protanomalous. (New London)
   - No report. Work continuing.

7. X-266
   - A field test of the ability of men with various degrees of anomaly to distinguish the color of signal lights at night. (New London)
   - No report. Work continuing.

8. X-347 - The critical hue regions of confusion of pigment colors under illuminant A and illuminant C for the color anomalous. (New London)

- No report. Work continuing.

9. X-348 - Retention of discriminable line at a distance for ten colors against the color of water. (New London)

- Report - (Preliminary) - RETENTION OF DISCRIMINABLE HUE OF TEN COLORS AT SMALL SUBTENSE, (Color Vision Report No. 7), 20 April 1944. (Farnsworth)

- Addendum Report - DIFFERENCES IN CHROMATIC DISCRIMINATION AT SMALL SUBTENSE, 22 April 1944. (Author unknown)

10. X-457 - Development and trial of New London Navy Lantern as a selection test for serviceable color vision. (New London)

- Report - (Preliminary) - A BRIEF HISTORY OF LANTERNS FOR TESTING COLOR SENSATION AND DESCRIPTION OF THE ESSENTIAL PRINCIPLES, 15 April 1946. (Farnsworth and Foreman)

- Report - (Final) - DEVELOPMENT AND TRIAL OF NEW LONDON NAVY LANTERN AS A SELECTION TEST FOR SERVICEABLE COLOR VISION, (COLOR VISION Report No. 12), 6 May 1946. (Farnsworth and Foreman)

11. X-480 - Comparison and evaluation of the "Pseudo-isochromatic plates for testing of Color Perception", American Optical Company, Second Edition, with the first edition of these plates now in general use by the U. S. Navy, Corpus Christi, Pensacola, Jacksonville, San Diego, New London, Norfolk, Camp Lejeune, and Alameda.

- Report - Same title as above, 30 December 1944. (Staff of the Medical Department, Corpus Christi)

- Report No. 1 - Same title as above, 21 November 1944. (Wolpaw and Imus) (Pensacola)

- Report - Same title as above, 15 February 1945. (Carter) (Jacksonville)

- Report - Same title as above, 16 January 1945. (Mueller) (San Diego)

- Report - Same title as above, COLOR VISION REPORT No. 8, 19 March 1945. (Farnsworth and Reed) (New London)

- Report - (First and Fiaal) - Same title as above, 16 July 1945. (Sulzman) (Norfolk)

- Report - Same title as above, 13 August 1945. (Ross and Mueller) (Camp Lejeune)

- Report - (Letter form) - Same title as above, 2 January 1945. (White) (Alameda)

12. X-502 - Effect of tinted lenses on color vision. (New London)

- Report - THE EFFECT OF COLORED LENSES UPON COLOR DISCRIMINATION, Color Vision Report No. 9, 3 September 1945. (Farnsworth)

13. X-613 - Development and Trial of screening devices for detection of anomalous color vision for use in ophthalmic instruments. (New London)

- No report. Work continuing.

VISION

Form I Vision Examination

1. X-395 - Evaluation of eye examination: NMSAv-Form I. (Pensacola)

   - No report. Work continuing.

Miscellaneous

1. X-149 - Changes in visual fields under stress of naval conditions. (NMRI)

   - Report No. 1 - MEASUREMENTS OF "VISUAL" FIELDS WITH THE PERIMETER UNDER CONDITIONS OF PHYSIOLOGIC STRESS, 26 November 1945. (Blum and Fisher)

2. X-170 - Photographic study of eye movements in instrument flying. (Atlanta)

   - Progress Report - Same title as above, August 1944. (McGehee)

   - Report - (Final) - TED NO. ATL-R 601; COMPARATIVE STUDY OF PILOT FATIGUE RESULTING FROM EXTENDED INSTRUMENT FLIGHT USING THE STANDARD AAF AND BRITISH INSTRUMENT PANELS. (McGehee) This study made for BuAer but covered the items in X-170 and served as report in this project.

3. X-290 - A study of marksmanship efficiency under conditions of low illumination. (Camp Lejeune)

   - Report - Same title as above, 1 July 1944. (Webster and Corey)

4. X-541 - Effect of gravitational force (tilt table) on alteration of scotopic vision and means of prevention of this effect. (Pensacola)

   - Report No. 1 - THE EFFECT UPON SCOTOPIC VISION OF CIRCULATORY CHANGES INDUCED BY NITROGLYCERINE AND CHANGE IN BODY POSITION, 22 March 1946. (Patterson, Burt, and Jones)

NIGHT VISION - DARK ADAPTATION

1. X-20 - Study of dark adaptation and ship's lighting. (USS Enterprise)

   - Report - DARK ADAPTATION STUDY, USS ENTERPRISE, 23 March 1942. (Weinbach)

2. X-22 - Development of specifications for dark adaptation goggles. (NIH)

   - Report - THE INFLUENCE OF BRIGHTNESS OF RED AND WHITE PREADAPTING LIGHTS ON THE COURSE OF DARK ADAPTATION FOR VARIOUS COLORS OF TEST FIELDS AND TESTS OF SPECIFIC GOGGLES SUBMITTED BY THE MEDICAL RESEARCH SECTION, BuAer, 25 March 1942. (Weinbach and Lee)

3. X-23 - Interrelationship of eyes in dark adaptation. (NIH)

   - Report - BINOCULAR ADAPTATION - THE INDEPENDENCE OF THE STATE OF ADAPTATION OF ONE EYE UPON THAT OF THE OTHER EYE, 30 January 1942. (Lee and Weinbach)

4. X-142 - Growth curve of light adaptation. (NIH)

   - Report - EXPLORATORY PROJECT ON GROWTH CURVE OF LIGHT ADAPTATION, 8 April 1943. (Lee)

5. X-162 - Determination of effect on dark adaptation of varying intensities of illumination in ready rooms. (NMRI and NIH)

   - Report No. 1 - (NMRI) - Same title as above, 2 June 1943. (Lee)

   - Report No. 2 - (NMRI) - DETERMINATION OF EFFECT ON DARK ADAPTATION OF VARYING INTENSITIES OF ILLUMINATION IN READY ROOMS: NEWLY DISCOVERED FLUCTUATIONS OF PERIODIC NATURE OCCURRING IN DARK ADAPTATION THRESHOLDS, 24 September 1943. (Lee, Fisher, and Birren)

6. X-196 - Effect of aircraft radar on dark adaptation. (NRL)

   - Report No. NRL H-2226 - EFFECT OF CATHODE RAY TUBE SCREENS ON NIGHT VISION, 31 January 1944. (Tousey)

7. X-211 - Investigation of rhythmic fluctuations appearing in dark adaptation curves and their influence on reliability of form perception tests. (NMRI and NIH)

- Report No. 1 - (NMRI) - A METHOD OF CURVE FITTING APPLICABLE TO DARK ADAPTATION AND SIMILAR DATA CONTAINING PERIODIC FLUCTUATIONS ABOUT A SMOOTH CURVE, 11 September 1944. (Lee and Finch)

- Report No. 2 - (NMRI) - PERIODIC FLUCTUATIONS AND THRESHOLD LEVELS IN DARK ADAPTATION AND THE EFFECTS PRODUCED BY PAREDRINE, OXYGEN, CARBON DIOXIDE, AND ASCORBIC ACID, 12 September 1944. (Lee, Pijoan, Catchpole, and Finch)

8. X-218 - Comparison of rates of dark adaptation under red illumination and in total darkness. (NMRI and NIH)

- Report - (NMRI) - Same title as above, 30 December 1943. (Lee)

9. X-254 - Determination of levels of illumination at which binocular fusion can take place. (NMRI)

- Report - A STUDY OF BINOCULAR FUSION AT LOW LEVELS OF ILLUMINATION, 25 May 1944. (Blum and Fisher)

10. X-351 - Rate of readaptation after exposure to white light. (Pensacola)

- Report - THE COURSE OF READAPTATION AFTER EXPOSURE TO WHITE LIGHT, 23 February 1944. (Peckham)

11. X-407 - Night vision tests on wired goggles (non-fogging). (NMRI)

- Report - Same title as above, 14 August 1944. (Lee and Finch)

12. X-439 - Orange Dark Adaptor Goggle. (Pensacola)

- Report No. 1 - THE COURSE OF DARK ADAPTATION AFTER WEARING ORANGE DARK ADAPTOR GOGGLES, 19 February 1945. (Clark and Johnson)

13. X-442 - Influence of exposure to intense sunlight on subsequent night vision. (Camp Lejeune)

- Preliminary Report - THE INFLUENCE OF SUNLIGHT ON NIGHT VISION CONTAINED IN MINUTES OF ARMY-NAVY-OSRD VISION COMMITTEE - 6th MEETING, 12 October 1944. (Hecht)

- Report - Same title as above, 26 April 1945. (Hecht, Hendley, Ross, and Richmond)

14. X-483

- The effectiveness of colored versus neutral dark adaptation goggles. (Anacostia)

- Report - Same title as above, December 1944. (Peckham and Older)

15. X-503

- Effect of searchlights on dark adaptation. (Quonset Point)

- Report No. 1 - THE EFFECT OF THE NAVY AIRBORNE SEARCHLIGHT ON DARK ADAPTATION, 2 May 1945. (Orlansky)

16. X-548

- Effect of long wavelength ultra-violet in the region between 3200 and 4000 angstrom units on dark adaptation. (NMRI)

- Report No. 1 - EFFECT OF SHORT EXPOSURES TO RADIATION FROM A LANDING SIGNAL OFFICER'S LAMP ON DARK ADAPTATION, 12 April 1945. (Lee)

17. NMRI-121 TED UNL 25184

- The effect on Dark Adaptation of the Fluorescent Material of Oxygen Flow Indicator, (DJ-2-1) (NMRI)

- Report - Same title as above, 26 May 1945. (Lee)

VISION

Night Vision Scotometry

1. X-492 - Trial of the Livingston Method of Rod Scotometry and Comparison of Results with Radium Plaque Adaptometer Scores. (Norfolk and New London)

   - Progress Report No. 1 - (New London) - A STUDY OF THE PHYSIOLOGICAL BLIND - SPOT OF THE DARK ADAPTED FOVEA, 1 March 1946. (Sulzman)

   - Work is continuing.

2. X-529 - Development of diaphragm shutter scotometer. (NMRI)

   - Report No. 1 - Same title as above, 18 July 1945. (Korb)

3. X-614 - An experimental evaluation of the Korb Diaphragm Scotometer as a test of Night Vision. (Quonset Point and New London)

   - Progress Report - (Quonset Point) - (Memorandum Form) - KORB DIAPHRAGM SCOTOMETER PROJECT, 19 June 1945. (Orlansky)

   - Progress Report No. 1 - (New London) - A STUDY OF THE PHYSIOLOGICAL BLIND - SPOT OF THE DARK-ADAPTED FOVEA, 1 March 1946. (Sulzman)

VISION

Night Vision Testing

1. X-24 - Hecht Adaptometer, Model 2: Determination of norms and test-retest reliability for. (Pensacola)

   - Status Report, 25 April 1942. (Author unknown)

   - Report - NIGHT VISION, ADAPTOMETERS FOR. TESTING AND METHODS OF ADMINISTERING TESTS, 6 May 1942. (Weinbach)

   - Report - (Progress) - RESEARCH PROJECT NIGHT VISION, 11 May 1942. (No author given)

   - Report in letter form; NIGHT VISION, TESTS OF, 6 June 1942. (Peckham)

2. X-25 - NDRC Adaptometer, Model 2: Determination of norms and test-retest reliability for. (Pensacola and New London)

   - Status Report - (Pensacola) - 25 April 1942. (Author unknown)

   - Report - NIGHT VISION, ADAPTOMETERS FOR. TESTING AND METHODS OF ADMINISTERING TESTS, 6 May 1942. (Weinbach)

   - Report - (Progress) - RESEARCH PROJECT NIGHT VISION, 11 May 1942. (No author given)

   - Report in letter form: NIGHT VISION, TESTS OF, 6 June 1942. (Peckham)

   - Report - (Letter form) - (New London - Board of Medical Examiners for Night Vision) RELIABILITY TEST OF N.D.R.C. ADAPTOMETER, MODEL II, 20 July 1942. (Shilling)

3. X-26 - Radium Plaque Adaptometer: Determination of norms and test-retest reliability for. (Pensacola)

   - Status Report - 25 April 1942. (Author unknown)

   - Report - NIGHT VISION, ADAPTOMETERS FOR. TESTING AND METHODS OF ADMINISTERING TESTS, 6 May 1942. (Weinbach)

- Report - (Progress) - RESEARCH PROJECT NIGHT VISION, 11 May 1942. (No author given)

- Report in letter form: NIGHT VISION, TESTS OF, 6 June 1942. (Peckham)

4. X-27

- Determination of Intercorrelations between test Scores on Hecht, NDRC and Radium Plaque Adaptometers. (Pensacola)

- Status Report - 25 April 1942. (Author unknown)

- Report - NIGHT VISION, ADAPTOMETERS FOR. TESTING AND METHODS OF ADMINISTERTING TESTS, 6 May 1942. (Weinbach)

- Report - (Progress) - RESEARCH PROJECT NIGHT VISION, 11 May 1942. (No author given)

- Report in letter form - NIGHT VISION, TESTS OF, 6 June 1942. (Peckham)

5. X-28

- Development of a Reliable Means for Scoring Actual Field Performance of Night Observers. (Pensacola)

- Status Report - 25 April 1942. (Author unknown)

- Report - NIGHT VISION, ADAPTOMETERS FOR TESTING AND METHODS OF ADMINISTERING TESTS, 6 May 1942. (Weinbach)

- Report - (Progress) - RESEARCH PROJECT NIGHT VISION, 11 May 1942. (No author given)

- Report in letter form - NIGHT VISION, TESTS OF, 6 June 1942. (Peckham)

6. X-29

- Correlation of Adaptometer Scores from Projects VI-5, 6, 7, 8, (X-24, X-25, X-26, X-27), with Actual Performance. (Pensacola and New London)

- Status Report - 25 April 1942. (Author unknown)

- Report - NIGHT VISION, ADAPTOMETERS FOR. TESTING AND METHODS OF ADMINISTERING TESTS, 6 May 1942. (Weinbach)

- Report - (Progress) - RESEARCH PROJECT NIGHT VISION, 11 May 1942. (No author given)

- Report in letter form: NIGHT VISION, TESTS OF, 6 June 1942. (Peckham)

7. X-31

- Night Sky Brightness. (Johnson Foundation, Univ. of Pennsylvania, and Pensacola)

- Status Report - 25 April 1942. (Author unknown)

- Report - NIGHT VISION, ADAPTOMETERS FOR. TESTING AND METHODS OF ADMINISTERING TESTS, 6 May 1942. (Weinbach)

- Report - (Progress) - RESEARCH PROJECT NIGHT VISION, 11 May 1942. (No author given)

- Report in letter form: NIGHT VISION, TESTS OF, 6 June 1942. (Peckham)

8. X-68

- Telesilhouette adaptometers, Self Luminous Type, Field Tests of. (New London)

- Report - COMPARATIVE STUDY OF ADAPTOMETERS, 1 December 1942. (Night Vision Board)

9. X-94

- Test-retest reliability of the adaptometer. (New London)

- Report in letter form - ADAPTOMETER - REPORT OF PROJECT X-94 (Av-V1-18) OF NOVEMBER 19,1942, TEST-RETEST RELIABILITY OF, 1 January 1943. (Beals,Jr.)

- Report - FURTHER REPORT ON THE TESTING OF EFFICIENCY OF NIGHT VISION: COMPARATIVE RELIABILITY AND VALIDITY MEASURES ON THE ADAPTOMETER AND THE SELF-LUMINOUS TELESILHOUETTE ADAPTOMETER, January 1943. (Beals and Verplanck)

10. X-137

- Test-retest of Wright adaptometer. (New London)

- Report - TEST-RETEST RELIABILITY OF THE WRIGHT ADAPTOMETER, March 1943. (Verplanck and Reed)

11. X-138

- Test-retest of Admiralty adaptometer, Mark I, No. 33. (New London)

- Report - TEST-RETEST RELIABILITY OF THE ADMIRALTY MARK I ADAPTOMETER, 1943. (Verplanck and Reed)

12. X-167

- Physical and physiological calibration of NDRC model III adaptometer. (NMRI, NIH, and New London)
- Report No. 1 - (NMRI) - Same title as above, 4 June 1943. (Lee and Fisher)
- Report - (Preliminary) - (New London) - NIGHT VISION TESTING OF THE CREW OF THE BATTLESHIP NEW JERSEY - A REPORT ON THE NDRC MODEL III ADAPTOMETER, 7 June 1943. (Verplanck)
- Report - (General) - NIGHT VISION TESTING OF MEMBERS OF THE CREW OF THE USS NEW JERSEY, 25 June 1943. (Verplanck)
- Report - NIGHT VISION TESTING OF MEMBERS OF THE CREW OF THE USS NEW JERSEY - INCIDENTAL DATA OF INTEREST, 3 July 1943. (Verplanck)

13. X-268

- Field test of Radium Plaque Adaptometer and of the instructions provided. (New London)
- Report - FIELD TESTS OF THE RADIUM PLAQUE ADAPTOMETER, 26 November 1943. (Verplanck, Watson, and Reed)
- Report - REPORT OF FIVE HUNDRED SUBJECTS TESTED AND RETESTED FOR FIFTY TRIALS EACH ON THE NAVY RADIUM PLAQUE ADAPTOMETER, 8 March 1944. (Peckham and Verplanck)
- Report - A REPORT ON THE NIGHT VISION TESTING OF 5,750 MEN, 12 August 1944. (Verplanck)
- Interval Report No. 3 - THE EFFECT OF INCREASING THE DIFFICULTY OF THE RPA TEST OF NIGHT VISION, 25 September 1945. (Verplanck)
- Work is continuing.

14. X-298

- Field Study of Navy Radium Plaque Adaptometer. (Corpus Christi)
- Report - Same title as above, 15 April 1944. (Macmillan and Commoner)

15. X-300 - Field Study of Navy Radium Plaque Adaptometer. (Annapolis)

- Report - Same title as above, 1 April 1944. (Wilson and Triedke)

16. X-311 - Design and construction of a portable multiple brightness Radium Plaque Adaptometer. (NMRI)

- Report No. 1 - DESIGN, CONSTRUCTION, AND PRELIMINARY EVALUATION OF A PORTABLE MULTIPLE BRIGHTNESS RADIUM PLAQUE ADAPTOMETER, 11 August 1945. (Draeger, Lee, and Fisher)

17. X-466 - Evaluation of new Radium Plaque Adaptometer (Modified Rostenberg Adaptometer) Constructed under Project N-115 of the Applied Psychology Panel, NDRC. (NMRI)

- Report - RECHECK FOR NIGHT BLINDNESS OF 115 OFFICER CANDIDATES AT THE NAVAL RESERVE MIDSHIPMEN SCHOOL, COLUMBIA UNIVERSITY, 18 December 1944. (Lee)

- Report No. 1 - EVALUATION OF THE MODIFIED ROSTENBERG ADAPTOMETER, 8 May 1945. (Lee and Fisher)

18. X-472 - An investigation of the effect of varying the test distance upon RPA scores. (Camp Lejeune)

- Progress Report No. 1 - Same title as above, 27 April 1945. (Ross)

- Progress Report No. 2 - Same title as above, 15 May 1945. (Ross)

- Progress Report No. 3 - Same title as above, 17 July 1945. (Ross and Mueller)

- Progress Report No. 4 - Same title as above, 21 November 1945. (Mueller, Richmond, and Ross)

VISION

Night Vision - Night Vision Training

1. X-558 - The effect of night vision training (Evelyn Trainer) on U. S. Navy Radium Plaque Adaptometer scores. (Quonset Point)

   - Report No. 1 - Same title as above, 16 April 1945. (Orlansky)

2. X-563 - A study of the learning resulting from the use of the Navy night vision training devices. (Pensacola)

   - Report No. 1 - Same title as above, 25 July 1945. (Clark, Nadel, Johnson and Dreher)

3. X-582 - The effect of night vision training on Radium Plaque Adaptometer test failure rate. (Camp Lejeune)

   - Report - THE EFFECT OF NIGHT VISION TRAINING ON R.P.A. TEST FAILURE RATE, 9 June 1945. (Ross and Mueller)

VISION

Miscellaneous

1. X-30 - The Preparation of an Educational Manual on the subject "The Use of the Eyes at Night". (BUMED)

- Manual entitled as above, 15 April 1942. (Liljencrantz, Swanson and Carson)

2. X-89 - Instruction syllabus for night seeing. (Pensacola)

- Report - NIGHT VISION INSTRUCTION REPORT, 22 February 1943. (No author given)

3. X-423 - Variations in visual acuity under conditions of low illumination. Possible use as selection procedure and in assignment to duty. (Harvard University and New London)

- No report - work is continuing.

4. X-467 - Investigation of peripheral field reduction in night vision. (NMRI)

- No report - work is continuing.

VISION

Optical Instruments

1. X-156 - Trial of binoculars with fixed diopter and inter-pupillary setting. (New London)

- Report - A REPORT ON SAMPLE BINOCULAR SERIAL #6268, Mark I, Model 2, 23 July 1943. (Shilling)

2. X-638 - A field test of the use of filters and goggles in penetrating haze. (New London)

- Report (Preliminary) - FIELD TESTS OF OPTICAL INSTRUMENTS, 25 February 1946. (Verplanck)

- Work is continuing.

3. X-662 - Field tests of optical instruments and auxiliary experiments. (New London)

- Report (Preliminary) - FIELD TESTS OF OPTICAL INSTRUMENTS, 25 February 1946. (Verplanck)

- Work is continuing.

VISION

Protection of Vision

1. X-172 - Laboratory test of anti-glare spectacles. (NMRI)

- Report No. 1 (Final) - Same title as above, 18 June 1943. (King and Birren)

2. X-173 - Field trial of Polarized antiglare spectacles. (Pensacola)

- Report No. 1 - Same title as above, 22 September 1943. (Peckham, King, West and Henry)

3. X-203 - Evaluation of fogging characteristics of the Polaroid X-29 aviation type goggle. (NMRI and Patuxent River)

- Report No. 1 - Same title as above, 31 August 1943. (Blum, Lee and White)

- Report X-203A - TESTING OF GOGGLES (TED No. UNL 2533) ELECTRICALLY HEATED SINGLE APERTURE TYPE - MANUFACTURED BY GENERAL ELECTRIC COMPANY, 30 December 1943. (Lee)

- Report - X-203B - FIELD TESTS ON POLAROID X-29 AVIATION TYPE GOGGLES, 4 April 1944. (King and Mathis)

4. X-276 TED UNL 2544 - Test of plastic inserts for aviator's goggles. (NMRI)

- Report - Same title as above, 12 June 1944. (Lee and Blum)

5. X-319 - Comparison of fusion density and variable density sun scanning goggles. (NMRI)

- Report - FUSION DENSITY SUN-SCANNING GOGGLES, 31 March 1944. (Blum)

6. X-321 - Comparison tests of fusion-density and variable density sun-scanning goggles. (Anacostia)

- Report in letter form. Same title as above, 14 March 1944. (Dunn)

7. X-456 - Computation of adequate sun-scanning device. (BUMED)

- Report - Same title as above, 5 November 1945. (Peckham)

8. X-464 - Firing tests of proposed shooting glasses. (Camp Lejeune)

- Report - Same title as above, 18 April 1945. (Ross and Williams)

9. X-542 - Study of the effectiveness of Glasses, Sun, N-1, Contract No. NXsX - 66844. (Camp Lejeune)

- No report - work is continuing.

10. X-561 - Study of the Effectiveness of Glasses, Sun, N-1, Contract No. NXsX - 66844. (Pensacola)

- Report No. 1 - A STUDY OF THE EFFECTIVENESS OF SUNGLASSES IN THE PROTECTION OF NIGHT VISION, 7 September 1945. (Clark, Johnson, and Dreher)

11. X-567 - Investigation of protection afforded by sunglasses to retinal sensitivity. (Pensacola)

- Report No. 1 - THE EFFECT OF EXCESSIVE SUNLIGHT ON THE RETINAL SENSITIVITY OF AN UNPROTECTED AND A COMPLETELY PROTECTED EYE IN THE SAME INDIVIDUAL, 11 August 1945. (Clark, Johnson and Dreher)

- Report No. 2 - THE PROTECTION TO NIGHT VISION AFFORDED BY SUNGLASSES, 18 October 1945. (Clark, Johnson and Dreher)

12. X-583 - A study of the durability of glasses, Sun, N-1, Contract No. NXsX - 66844. (Camp Lejeune)

- Report - A STUDY OF THE DURABILITY OF GLASSES, SUN, N-1, Contract No. NXsX - 66844, 27 August 1945. (Ross and Mueller)

VISION

Radiant Energy

1. X-435 - Preparation of a standard curve for maximum expected intensity of sunlight at the retina. (NMRI)

   - Report - SOLAR ENERGY REACHING THE RETINA: PROPOSED SPECTRAL CURVE FOR TESTING SUN-SCANNING GLASSES, 1 August 1944. (Blum)

2. X-453 - Computation of ultraviolet and infrared intensity on certain airplane plastic windows. (BUMED)

   - Report - Same title as above, 5 November 1945. (Peckham)

3. X-648 TED UNL 25141 - Goggles, non-fluorescent. (USS CHARGER)

   - Report - TED No. UNL 25141.2 - GOGGLES, NON-FLUORESCENT, FOR USE BY LANDING SIGNAL OFFICERS WITH FLUORESCENT SUITS - TESTS OF. (Date and author unknown)

4. X-658 - Study of landing signal officer's equipment for night use. (NMRI)

   - No reports - work is continuing.

VISION

Stereoscopic Vision

1. X-33 - Vectographic test of stereoscopic vision and correlation with other depth perception tests. (Philadelphia)

- Memorandum Report - THREE DIMENSIONAL CORPORATION TEST, October 1942. (Pfaffman)

- Report - AN EXPERIMENTAL STUDY OF DEPTH PERCEPTION IN LANDING AIRPLANES, March 1943. (Pfaffman)

2. X-130 - Stromberg-Gwathmey test of depth perception - Cross Validation of. (Anacostia and New Orleans)

- Report - THE VALIDATION OF THE GWATHMEY-STROMBERG TEST OF DEPTH PERCEPTION, December 1942. (USNRAB, New Orleans)

- Report (Final) - Same title as above, 29 November 1945. (Fontaine and Channel)

3. X-717 - The Reliability of the Verhoeff test of Depth Perception. (Pensacola)

- Report No. 1 - Same title as above, 3 May 1946. (Trumbull)

VISION

Vision Testing

1. X-468 - Comparison of industrial testing device with Snellen chart and phorometer. (Pensacola)

   - Report No. 1 - Same title as above, 8 November 1944. (Wolpaw and Imus)

2. X-471 - Comparative study of screening devices for visual selection of naval personnel. (Camp Lejeune)

   - No report - work is continuing.

3. X-493 - Comparison of various screening devices with standard medical procedure. (New London)

   - Report (Second Preliminary) - COMPARISON OF VARIOUS SCREENING DEVICES WITH STANDARD MEDICAL PROCEDURE, 27 April 1945. (Sulzman, Farnsworth, Bartlett and Kindred)

   - Progress Report No. 1 - Same title as above, November 1945. (Sulzman, Farnsworth, Cook, Bartlett and Kindred)

   - Progress Report No. 2 - VISUAL ACUITY MEASUREMENTS WITH THREE COMMERCIAL SCREENING DEVICES, 7 February 1946. (Sulzman, Cook and Bartlett)

   - Progress Report No. 3 - COMPARATIVE STUDY OF MEASURES OF HETEROPHORIA, 22 February 1946. (Sulzman, Cook and Bartlett)

4. X-499 - Comparison of Orthorater with clinical ophthalmic examinations. (Pensacola)

   - Report No. 1 - Same title as above, 29 September 1945. (Wolpaw and Imus)

   - Report No. 2 - Same title as above, 1 March 1946. (Imus)

5. X-671 - Study of visual acuity targets. (Camp Lejeune)

   - No report - work is continuing.

6. X-672 - The effect of glasses, Sun, N-1, on visual acuity at high brightness. (Camp Lejeune)

- No report - work is continuing.

7. X-676 - A comparison of the reliability and validity of visual acuity test targets. (Pensacola)

- Report No. 1 - Same title as above, 3 April 1946. (Trumbull and Backstrom)

Made in United States
Troutdale, OR
11/03/2026

56852687R00100